T0214641

# Lecture Notes in Computer Science    11404

Commenced Publication in 1973
Founding and Former Series Editors:
Gerhard Goos, Juris Hartmanis, and Jan van Leeuwen

More information about this series at http://www.springer.com/series/7412

Tomaž Vrtovec · Jianhua Yao
Guoyan Zheng · Jose M. Pozo (Eds.)

# Computational Methods and Clinical Applications in Musculoskeletal Imaging

6th International Workshop, MSKI 2018
Held in Conjunction with MICCAI 2018
Granada, Spain, September 16, 2018
Revised Selected Papers

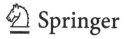 Springer

*Editors*
Tomaž Vrtovec
University of Ljubljana
Ljubljana, Slovenia

Guoyan Zheng
University of Bern
Bern, Switzerland

Jianhua Yao
Tencent
Shenzhen, China

Jose M. Pozo
University of Leeds
Leeds, UK

ISSN 0302-9743          ISSN 1611-3349   (electronic)
Lecture Notes in Computer Science
ISBN 978-3-030-11165-6          ISBN 978-3-030-11166-3   (eBook)
https://doi.org/10.1007/978-3-030-11166-3

Library of Congress Control Number: 2018966327

LNCS Sublibrary: SL6 – Image Processing, Computer Vision, Pattern Recognition, and Graphics

This Springer imprint is published by the registered company Springer Nature Switzerland AG
The registered company address is: Gewerbestrasse 11, 6330 Cham, Switzerland

# Preface

The musculoskeletal system consists of the skeleton, muscles, cartilage, ligaments, joints, and other connective tissue that supports and binds tissues and organs together, and provides form, support, protection, stability, and movement to the body. Specific subsystems like the spine provide both a vital central axis for the musculoskeletal system and a flexible protective shell surrounding the most important neural pathway in the body, the spinal cord. The musculoskeletal system is involved in various disease processes associated with aging and degeneration of bones and joints, such as osteoporosis and osteoarthritis. Osteoporosis is a condition where bones become brittle and fragile from loss of tissue due to hormonal changes, or deficiency in calcium or vitamin D. Osteoporosis leads to an increased bone fracture risk, which is further exacerbated in the elderly owing to the loss of muscular strength and frailty. Osteoarthritis, or degenerative arthritis, is caused by inflammation and the eventual loss of cartilage in the joints, which wears down with time. These are just a few relevant examples of the conditions associated with the musculoskeletal system, not to mention therapeutic procedures in orthopedic surgery, and the related medical implants and devices where imaging plays a crucial role in the planning, guidance, and monitoring phases. As a specialty of diagnostic radiology, musculoskeletal imaging involves the acquisition, analysis, and interpretation of medical images of bones, joints, and associated soft tissues for injury and disease diagnosis and treatment. Given the increasing volume of multimodal imaging examinations associated with musculoskeletal diseases and the complexity of their assessment, there is a pressing need for advanced computational methods that support diagnosis, therapy planning, and interventional guidance, with several related challenges in both methodology and clinical applications.

The goal of the workshop series on Computational Methods and Clinical Applications in Musculoskeletal Imaging is to bring together clinicians, researchers, and industrial vendors in musculoskeletal imaging for reviewing the state-of-the-art techniques, sharing novel and emerging analysis and visualization techniques, and discussing the clinical challenges and open problems in this field. Topics of interest include all major aspects of musculoskeletal imaging, for example: clinical applications of musculoskeletal computational imaging; computer-aided detection and diagnosis of conditions of the bones, muscles, and joints; image-guided musculoskeletal surgery and interventions; image-based assessment and monitoring of surgical and pharmacological treatment; segmentation, registration, detection, localization, and visualization of the musculoskeletal anatomy; statistical and geometrical modeling of the musculoskeletal shape and appearance; image-based microstructural characterization of musculoskeletal tissue; novel techniques for musculoskeletal imaging.

The 6th Workshop on Computational Methods and Clinical Applications in Musculoskeletal Imaging, MICCAI-MSKI2018[1], was a half-day satellite event of the 21st International Conference on Medical Image Computing and Computer-Assisted Intervention, MICCAI 2018[2], held during September 16–20, 2018, in Granada, Spain. The workshop was a continuation of the former Workshop on Computational Methods and Clinical Applications for Spine Imaging, CSI, which was, after four successful consecutive editions at MICCAI 2013, 2014, 2015, and 2016, opened up within its MICCAI-MSKI2017 edition to a wider community by broadening the scope from spine to musculoskeletal imaging, thereby recognizing the progress made in spine imaging and the emerging needs in imaging of other bones, joints, and muscles of the musculoskeletal system that was continued also in this year within MICCAI-MSKI 2018. We received several high-quality submissions addressing many of the aforementioned issues. All papers underwent a double-blind review, with each paper being reviewed by three members of the Review Committee. We finally accepted 13 out of 16 submitted papers, which were collected in soft-copy electronic proceedings distributed at the workshop and during the conference.

MICCAI-MSKI2018 was held on September 16, 2018, with the program consisting of three oral sessions: (1) Muscles and Bone Structures (three presentations), (2) Teeth, Wrist, Shoulder, and Ribs (four presentations), and (3) Hip and Pelvis (six presentations). To gain deeper insight into the field of musculoskeletal imaging and stimulating further ideas, an invited talk entitled "Multidisciplinary Computational Anatomy Modeling of Musculoskeletal Structures and Total Hip Arthroplasty from Medical Images" was given by Dr. Yoshinobu Sato from the Nara Institute of Science and Technology, Japan. The members of the Organizing Committee selected one outstanding contribution for the MICCAI-MSKI2018 Best Paper Award, which was given to the paper entitled "Deep Learning Based Rib Centerline Extraction and Labeling" by Matthias Lenga et al. from Philips Research Europe, Germany. After the workshop, the authors were invited to revise and resubmit their papers by considering the comments of the reviewers and the eventual feedback from the workshop itself, to be considered for publication in Springer's *Lecture Notes in Computer Science* (LNCS) series. The authors of all 13 papers presented at the workshop responded to the call, and after reviewing the resubmitted papers, the members of the Organizing Committee agreed that the revisions were of adequate quality, thus the papers now appear, in the chronological order of the initial submission, in these LNCS proceedings.

We would like to thank everyone who contributed to this workshop: the authors for their contributions, the members of the Program and Review Committee for their review work, promotion of the workshop, and general support, the invited speaker for sharing his expertise and knowledge, and the MICCAI Society for the opportunity to

---

[1] https://mski2018.wordpress.com.

[2] https://www.miccai2018.org.

exchange research ideas and build the community during the premier conference in medical imaging. Finally, we would like to invite the community to support the MSKI workshop in its future editions.

December 2018

Tomaž Vrtovec
Jianhua Yao
Guoyan Zheng
Jose M. Pozo

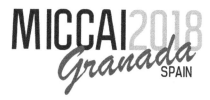
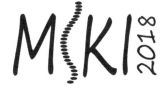

# Organization

## Program Chairs

| | |
|---|---|
| Tomaž Vrtovec | University of Ljubljana, Slovenia |
| Jianhua Yao | Tencent, China |
| Guoyan Zheng | University of Bern, Switzerland |
| Jose M. Pozo | The University of Sheffield and University of Leeds, UK |

## Program and Review Committee

| | |
|---|---|
| Ulas Bagci | University of Central Florida, USA |
| Paul A. Bromiley | The University of Manchester, UK |
| Weidong Cai | The University of Sydney, Australia |
| Daniel Forsberg | Sectra and Linköping University, Sweden |
| Huiguang He | The Chinese Academy of Sciences, China |
| Bulat Ibragimov | Auris Health and Stanford School of Medicine, USA |
| Samuel Kadoury | Polytechnique Montréal, Canada |
| Robert Korez | University of Ljubljana, Slovenia |
| Yoshito Otake | Nara Institute of Science and Technology, Japan |
| Greg Slabaugh | City, University of London, UK |
| Darko Štern | LBI CFI, Austria |
| Sovira Tan | National Institutes of Health, USA |
| Tamas Ungi | Queen's University, Canada |
| Qian Wang | Shanghai Jiao Tong University, China |
| Yiqiang Zhan | Shanghai Jiao Tong University, China |

## Proceedings Editors

| | |
|---|---|
| Tomaž Vrtovec | University of Ljubljana, Slovenia |
| Jianhua Yao | Tencent, China |
| Guoyan Zheng | University of Bern, Switzerland |
| Jose M. Pozo | The University of Sheffield and University of Leeds, UK |

# Contents

# Automated Recognition of Erector Spinae Muscles and Their Skeletal Attachment Region via Deep Learning in Torso CT Images

Naoki Kamiya[1(✉)], Masanori Kume[2], Guoyan Zheng[3], Xiangrong Zhou[4],
Hiroki Kato[5], Huayue Chen[6], Chisako Muramatsu[4], Takeshi Hara[4],
Toshiharu Miyoshi[7], Masayuki Matsuo[8], and Hiroshi Fujita[4]

[1] School of Information Science and Technology, Aichi Prefecture University,
Nagakute, Japan
n-kamiya@ist.aichi-pu.ac.jp
[2] Graduate School of National Science and Technology, Gifu University,
Gifu, Japan
[3] Institute for Surgical Technology and Biomechanics, University of Bern,
Bern, Switzerland
[4] Department of Electrical, Electronic and Computer Engineering, Gifu University,
Gifu, Japan
[5] Department of Radiology Service, Gifu University Hospital, Gifu, Japan
[6] School of Medicine, University of Occupational and Environmental Health,
Kitakyushu, Japan
[7] Radiology Service, Gifu University Hospital, Gifu, Japan
[8] Graduate School of Medicine, Department of Radiology, Gifu University,
Gifu, Japan

**Abstract.** Erector spinae muscle (ESM) is an important muscle in the torso region. Changes of sizes, shapes and densities in the cross section of the spinal column muscles have been found in chronic low back pain, degenerative lumbar sclerosis and chronic obstructive pulmonary disease. However, the image features of the ESM are measured manually by the physician. Therefore, automatic recognition in three dimensions (3D) not only for the limited two-dimensional (2D) section but also for the whole ESM is required. In this study, we realize automatic recognition of the ESMs and its attachment region on the skeleton using a 2D deep convolutional neural network. Each cross section of the 3D computed tomography (CT) image is input as a 2D image to the fully convolutional network. Then, the obtained result is reconstructed into a 3D image to obtain the recognition result of the ESM and its attachment region on the skeleton. ESM and attached area are extracted manually from the CT images of 11 cases and used for evaluation. In the experiments, automatic recognition was performed for each case using the leave-one-out method. The mean recognition accuracy of ESM and attached area was 89.9% and 65.5%, respectively for the Dice coefficient. In this study, although there is over-extraction in the recognition of the attachment region, the

© Springer Nature Switzerland AG 2019
T. Vrtovec et al. (Eds.): MSKI 2018, LNCS 11404, pp. 1–10, 2019.
https://doi.org/10.1007/978-3-030-11166-3_1

initial region has been acquired successfully and it is the first study to simultaneously recognize the ESMs and its attachment region on the skeleton.

**Keywords:** Erector spinae muscles · Skeletal muscles
Deep convolutional neural networks · Fully convolutional networks

# 1  Introduction

Erector spinae muscles (ESMs) are important muscles acting on extension and rotation at the trunk. In the chronic low back pain and the degenerative lumbar scoliosis (DLS), changes of the size, shape and density of the cross-sectional area (CSA) of the ESMs are found [1,2]. Furthermore, in the chronic obstructive pulmonary disease, the cross sectional area of the ESMs of the 12th thoracic vertebra is an excellent prognostic factor [3]. However, image analysis of these spinal column erector muscles is performed manually by clinicians. Therefore, the measurements suffer from inter-clinician reliability and intra-clinician reproducibility. In addition, spinal erector muscle is relatively large and has many adjacent muscles, extraction requires expertise and time consuming manual work. For these reasons, the current analysis remains limited to two-dimensional (2D) CSA, and investigation of the relationship between muscle and disease using three-dimensional (3D) area of ESM has not been realized.

Automatic recognition of skeletal muscle using computed tomography (CT) images is divided into 2D and 3D based methods. Wei et al. [4] realized the atlas based method to recognize the ESM automatically. In addition, there is automatic recognition method of skeletal muscle using finite element method (FEM) [5]. We proposed a deep convolutional neural network (CNN) based method to automatically recognize the ESM in the 12th thoracic section and obtained an average Jaccard coefficient (JC) of 82.4% [6]. On the other hand, in the method based on 3D, the goal is to obtain a 3D region of skeletal muscle. We created a computational anatomical model imitating muscle running and realized automatic recognition of surface parts [7] and deep muscles [8]. Moreover, in the automatic recognition method of ESM using random forest, the average Dice coefficient (DC) was $93.0 \pm 2.1\%$ [9]. In addition, Yokota et al. [10] realized automatic recognition of skeletal muscle in hip and femoral region by hierarchical multi-atlas method.

Analysis of diseases associated with the ESM [1–3] requires extracting a section corresponding to the level of the medullary node of the vertebrae. Furthermore, recognition of the anatomical attachment position of the skeletal muscle is important for generation of a computed anatomical model on the CT image and appropriate utilization of the model. Actually, in the creation of a muscle running model, the origin and insertion of each muscle is used [7,8]. In addition, in recognition of skeletal muscle at the shoulder part, recognition accuracy was improved by utilizing the structural features of the scapula which is the attachment part of the muscle in model building [11]. Therefore, recognition of the anatomical attachment position information on the muscle on the skeleton is necessary for construction and utilization of the model, analysis of the relationship between muscle and disease, as well as muscle recognition.

In this study using 2D-deep CNN, we aim to acquire not only muscle recognition results, but also regional information of origin and insertion which becomes attachment area on the skeleton which is necessary for muscle analysis.

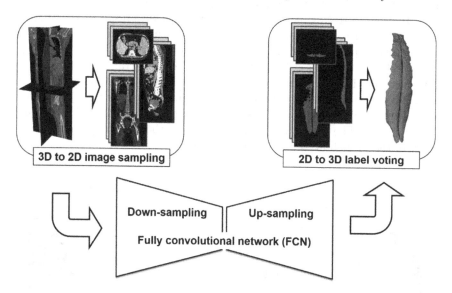

**Fig. 1.** A network of automatic recognition of erector spinae muscle and its attached areas on the skeleton. In three-dimensional (3D) to two-dimensional (2D) image sampling, each section is extracted from the computed tomography image as input images. In 2D to 3D label voting, recognition results of each section are integrated into a 3D image. Details of the fully convolutional network are described in Fig. 2.

## 2    Method

### 2.1    Overview

The proposed method is based on the automatic recognition method of multiple organs in 3D CT images using deep CNN [12]. The outline of this method is shown in Fig. 1. The input image is a torso CT image, and the output image is a label image of the spinal column erector muscle and the attached region on the skeleton. First, 2D images of three anatomical sections are obtained from input CT images. Thereafter, each 2D cross-sectional image is input to deep CNN, and region recognition is performed on each 2D cross-sectional image. Finally, recognition results in each obtained cross section are integrated as 3D images using label probabilities. A fully convolutional network (FCN) [13] is used for region recognition in the 2D section. In the training process in FCN, a CT image and a ground truth image obtained by extracting ESM and attachment areas on the skeleton of the ESM are used.

## 2.2  3D to 2D Image Sampling and 2D to 3D Label Voting

In our proposed method, 2D cross-sectional images are generated from 3D CT images as input images. Then, the ESM which is a target region in the 2D cross section and its attached region are recognized, and finally the recognition result in each cross section is reconstructed into a 3D image. It should be noted that each voxel on the 3D CT image belongs to a plurality of 2D cross-sectional images. In other words, by recognizing a target region with respect to a 2D image of a plurality of cross sections, it is aimed at enhancing recognition accuracy by performing label prediction a plurality of times for each voxel. Here, 2D images of three orthogonal cross sections, axial, coronal and sagittal, are created. As a result, each voxel is always arranged in three 2D images. After region recognition using 2D images, each voxel obtains three recognition results for each section. The result of recognition of each section is integrated into a 3D image using majority voting. The final label is determined by the maximum value of the product of the probabilities of each cross section.

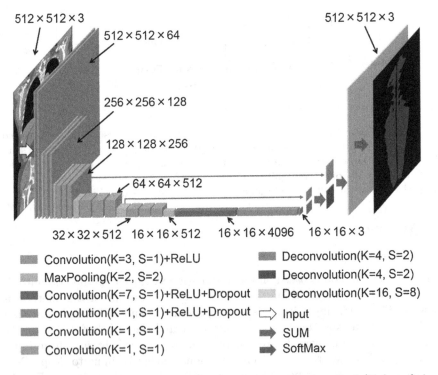

**Fig. 2.** Fully convolutional network structure of our proposed method (K: kernel size, S: stride).

## 2.3   ESM and Its Attachment Region Segmentation Using FCN

In this method, FCN is used in order to perform region recognition in 2D images of each section generated from a 3D image. The structure of FCN is composed of two layers, which are down sampling layer and up sampling layer, respectively. First, abstract information is extracted in the down sampling layer, and in the latter half of the up sampling layer, labels are predicted in pixel units. Each parameter of FCN is optimized by learning.

Figure 2 shows the FCN structure used in the proposed method. The down sampling layer consists of sixteen $3 \times 3$ convolution layers, five pooling layers and three full connected layers based on the network structure of VGG 16 [14]. In the FCN, the full connected layer in VGG 16 is replaced by a convolution layer. The last $1 \times 1$ convolution layer sets the number of labels classified channels. In this method, it is the three regions of the background, the ESM and its attachment region on the skeleton. The up sampling layer is composed of three deconvolution layers and two convolution layer. This network has a skip structure that uses the information lost in the convolution layer of the VGG 16 in the deconvolution layer. The network with one deconvolution layer is called FCN-32s and learning of FCN is repeated with the addition of deconvolution layer to construct FCN-16s, FCN-8s. In this method, the output of FCN-8s is taken as the recognition result of the 2D image. The activation function uses a rectified linear unit (ReLU).

## 2.4   Input Label Image

In the learning process of the network, the original image and the ground truth image are used. For the ground truth image, manually segmented images are used. An example of the ground truth image is shown in Fig. 3. Figure 3(a) shows the whole ESM in a 3D representation. A pair of the muscles are present on both sides of the body. The middle diagram shows the attachment area on the skeleton. Here, in the dorsal side of the ribs and the transverse process of the thoracic vertebra, the area on the skeleton which is in attached with the muscle is defined as the ground truth. This corresponds to the origin and insertion of the iliopsoas muscle and the longissimus muscle among the muscles constituting the ESM. In the learning process, the ESM and the attachment region on the skeleton are learned at the same time. Figure 3(b) shows a cross section where the ground truth on the original CT.

# 3   Experiment

CT images used in this study are non-contrast torso CT images taken by Light Speed Ultra 16 (manufactured by General Electric) at Gifu University Hospital, Japan. All the data have an isotropic voxel resolution of 0.625 mm. The size of the data ranges from $512 \times 512 \times 802$ voxels to $512 \times 512 \times 1031$ voxels. Eleven cases were used for the experiment and evaluated by the leave-one-out method. In learning, we used VGG 16's model trained with ImageNet ILSVRC-2014 data set [14] as a preliminary learning model. The DC, JC, recall rate and precision rate are used to evaluate recognition results of spinal column erector muscle and attached region on the skeleton.

For the implementation environment, the GPU uses 12 GB of NVIDIA GeForce TITAN - X, and the framework uses Caffe.

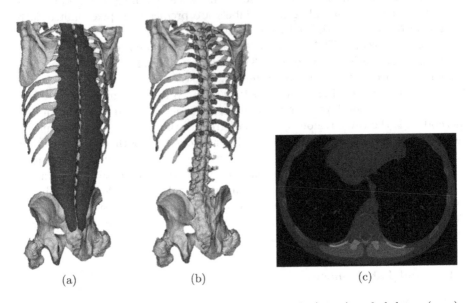

(a)                    (b)                    (c)

**Fig. 3.** Ground truth image. (a) Erector spinae muscle (green) and skeleton (gray). (b) Muscle attachment region on the skeleton (red). (c) Erector spinae muscle (green) and its attachment region on the skeleton (red). (Color figure online)

## 4   Results

Recognition results of ESMs in 11 cases are shown in Table 1. The mean JC of ESM recognition result was $81.7 \pm 3.2\%$, and the average DC was $89.9 \pm 2.0\%$. The average JC of recognition results of the ESM on the twelfth thoracic vertebra section was $85.6 \pm 3.7\%$, and the average DC was $92.2 \pm 2.2\%$. In addition, Table 2 shows the recognition result of the attachment region on the skeleton. The average JC of the recognition result of the attachment area on the skeleton was $48.8 \pm 3.7\%$, and the average DC was $65.5 \pm 3.3\%$. Figure 4 shows an example of the recognition result in 2D, and Fig. 5 shows the recognition result in 3D.

## 5   Discussion

The automatic recognition result of the ESM using 2D-deep CNN achieved an average DC of $89.9 \pm 2.0\%$. The achieved accuracy is slightly worse than that achieved by our random forest based ESM recognition method [9]. Although

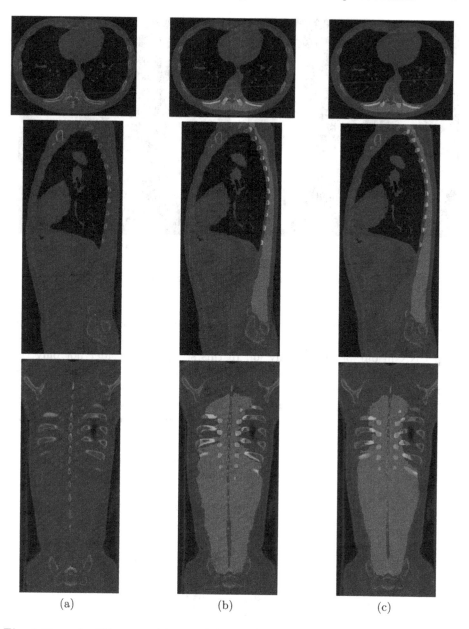

(a)                              (b)                              (c)

**Fig. 4.** Example of the recognition result in two-dimensional cross sections. (a) Original computed tomography images. (b) Ground truth images. (c) Recognition results.

both methods used the same training dataset, we attribute the less accurate results to the fact that deep CNN requires more learning cases as compared with conventional machine learning methods. On the other hand, the mean JC in the 12th thoracic vertebral section of this method was $85.6 \pm 3.7\%$. This is a high

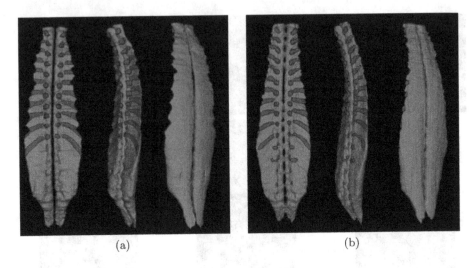

(a)                                        (b)

**Fig. 5.** (a) Ground truth. (b) Recognition result.

recognition accuracy compared with the average Jaccard coefficient of 82.4% in the automatic recognition method of the ESM in the 12th thoracic section using deep CNN in our previous study [6]. In this study, we consider not only the learning of the axial cross section but also the sagittal and the coronal sections, so in large skeletal muscle such as the ESM, learning process using both coronal and sagittal section is effective. Although the numerical value of the muscle attachment accuracy is low, as shown in Figs. 4 and 5, the origin and insertion

**Table 1.** Recognition result of the erector spinae muscles (JC: Jaccard coefficient, DC: Dice coefficient, RC: recall rate, PR: precision rate).

| Case | JC (%) | DC (%) | RC (%) | PR (%) |
|---|---|---|---|---|
| #1 | 84.1 | 91.4 | 91.6 | 91.1 |
| #2 | 82.0 | 90.1 | 89.9 | 90.2 |
| #3 | 85.0 | 91.9 | 91.7 | 92.1 |
| #4 | 74.5 | 85.4 | 79.6 | 92.1 |
| #5 | 81.5 | 89.8 | 95.6 | 84.7 |
| #6 | 84.5 | 91.6 | 92.9 | 90.3 |
| #7 | 83.9 | 91.2 | 95.8 | 87.1 |
| #8 | 77.9 | 87.6 | 96.8 | 79.9 |
| #9 | 84.4 | 91.5 | 94.2 | 89.0 |
| #10 | 80.8 | 89.4 | 94.7 | 84.6 |
| #11 | 80.3 | 89.1 | 97.9 | 81.7 |
| Average | 81.7 ± 3.2 | 89.9 ± 2.0 | 92.8 ± 5.0 | 87.5 ± 4.3 |

region is well recognized. The anatomical attachment site of skeletal muscle is one of the essential elements for orthopedic intervention and is important as well as recognition of skeletal muscle region.

**Table 2.** Recognition results of the erector spinae muscle attachment region on the skeleton (JC: Jaccard coefficient, DC: Dice coefficient, RC: recall rate, PR: precision rate).

| JC (%) | DC (%) | RC (%) | PR (%) |
|---|---|---|---|
| $48.8 \pm 3.7$ | $65.5 \pm 3.3$ | $72.6 \pm 10.3$ | $61.4 \pm 7.6$ |

In the next step, it is necessary to conduct a large-scale experiment with an increased number of cases and to verify the ESM recognition accuracy in deep CNN. However, it is not easy to create many ground truth of large and complex skeletal muscles such as the ESM. Therefore, it is necessary to efficiently generate a learning image in deep CNN by using our method using high speed and high performance random forest [9].

## 6   Conclusion

In this study, automatic recognition of ESMs and its attachment region on the skeleton in torso CT image by using deep CNN was performed. As a result of the leave-one-out cross validation test using eleven cases, the average Dice coefficient of ESM was $89.9 \pm 2.0\%$. In the 12th thoracic vertebra, the mean Jaccard coefficient was $85.6 \pm 3.7\%$. This result shows that automatic recognition is realized with high coincidence ratio in clinically important two-dimensional cross section, and it is a result that enables quantitative analysis by 3D. Although numerical recognition accuracy was low, simultaneous automatic recognition of the skeletal muscle and its anatomical attachment site, origin and insertion, was realized. For future work, we aim to clarify the relationship of 3D ESM using the recognized muscle region and its attachment position on the skeleton.

**Acknowledgements.** This research was supported in part by a Grant-in-Aid for Scientific Research on Innovative Areas (Grant No. 26108005 and 17H05301), MEXT, Japan.

## References

1. Danneels, L., Vanderstraeten, G., Cambier, D., Witvrouw, E., De Cuyper, H., Danneels, L.: CT imaging of trunk muscles in chronic low back pain patients and healthy control subjects. Eur. Spine J. **9**(4), 266–272 (2000). https://doi.org/10.1007/s005860000190

2. Yagi, M., Hosogane, N., Watanabe, K., Asazuma, T., Matsumoto, M.: The paravertebral muscle and psoas for the maintenance of global spinal alignment in patient with degenerative lumbar scoliosis. Spine J. **16**(4), 451–458 (2016). https://doi.org/10.1016/j.spinee.2015.07.001

3. Tanimura, K., et al.: Quantitative assessment of erector spinae muscles in patients with chronic obstructive pulmonary disease. Novel chest computed tomography-derived index for prognosis. Ann. Am. Thorac. Soc. **13**(3), 334–341 (2016). https://doi.org/10.1513/AnnalsATS.201507-446OC

4. Wei, Y., Xu, B., Tao, X., Qu, J.: Paraspinal muscle segmentation in CT images using a single atlas. In: Proceedings of IEEE International Conference on Progress in Informatics and Computing – PIC 2015, pp. 211–215. IEEE (2015). https://doi.org/10.1109/PIC.2015.7489839

5. Popuri, K., Cobzas, D., Esfandiari, N., Baracos, V., Jägersand, M.: Body composition assessment in axial CT images using FEM-based automatic segmentation of skeletal muscle. IEEE Trans. Med. Imaging **35**(2), 512–520 (2016). https://doi.org/10.1109/TMI.2015.2479252

6. Kume, M., et al.: Automated recognition of the erector spinae muscle based on deep CNN at the level of the twelfth thoracic vertebrae in torso CT images. In: Proceedings of 36th JAMIT Annual Meeting, pp. 74–76 (2017)

7. Kamiya, N., et al.: Automated segmentation of recuts abdominis muscle using shape model in X-ray CT images. In: Proceedings of 33rd Annual International Conference of the IEEE Engineering in Medicine and Biology Society – EMBC 2011, pp. 7993–7996. IEEE (2011). https://doi.org/10.1109/IEMBS.2011.6091971

8. Kamiya, N., et al.: Automated segmentation of psoas major muscle in X-ray CT images by use of a shape model: preliminary study. Radiol. Phys. Technol. **5**(1), 5–14 (2012). https://doi.org/10.1007/s12194-011-0127-0

9. Kamiya, N., Li, J., Kume, M., Fujita, H., Shen, D., Zheng, G.: Fully automatic segmentation of paraspinal muscles from 3D torso CT images via multi-scale iterative random forest classifications. In: Proceedings of 32nd International Congress and Exhibition on Computer Assisted Radiology and Surgery - CARS 2018, pp. 18–00047 (2018)

10. Yokota, F., et al.: Automated muscle segmentation from CT images of the hip and thigh using a hierarchical multi-atlas method. Int. J. Comput. Assist. Radiol. Surg. **13**(7), 977–986 (2018). https://doi.org/10.1007/s11548-018-1758-y

11. Katafuchi, T., et al.: Improvement of supraspinatus muscle recognition methods based on the anatomical features on the scapula in torso CT image. In: Proceedings of International Forum on Medical Imaging in Asia - IFMIA, pp. 315–316 (2017)

12. Zhou, X., Ito, T., Takayama, R., Wang, S., Hara, T., Fujita, H.: Three-dimensional CT image segmentation by combining 2D fully convolutional network with 3D majority voting. In: Carneiro, G., et al. (eds.) LABELS/DLMIA -2016. LNCS, vol. 10008, pp. 111–120. Springer, Cham (2016). https://doi.org/10.1007/978-3-319-46976-8_12

13. Long, J., Shelhamer, E., Darrell, T.: Fully convolutional networks for semantic segmentation. In: Proceedings of IEEE Conference on Computer Vision and Pattern Recognition – CVPR 2015, pp. 3431–3440. IEEE (2015). https://doi.org/10.1109/CVPR.2015.7298965

14. Simonyan, K., Zisserman, A.: Very deep convolutional networks for large-scale image recognition. arXiv:1409.1556 (2015)

# Fully Automatic Teeth Segmentation in Adult OPG Images

Nicolás Vila Blanco[1]([⊠]), Timothy F. Cootes[2], Claudia Lindner[2],
Inmaculada Tomás Carmona[3], and Maria J. Carreira[1]

[1] Centro de Investigación en Tecnoloxías da Información (CITIUS),
University of Santiago de Compostela, Santiago de Compostela, Spain
`nicolas.vila@usc.es`
[2] Centre for Imaging Sciences, University of Manchester, Manchester, UK
[3] Oral Sciences Research Group, Health Research Institute Foundation of Santiago de
Compostela, University of Santiago de Compostela, Santiago de Compostela, Spain

**Abstract.** This work addresses the problem of segmenting teeth in
panoramic dental images. Random forest regression voting constrained
local models were applied firstly to locate the mandible and the approximate pose of each tooth, and secondly to locate the full outline of
each individual tooth. An automatically computed quality-of-fit measure was proposed to identify missing teeth. The system was evaluated
using 346 manually annotated images containing adult-stage mandibular teeth. Encouraging results were achieved for detecting missing teeth.
The system achieved state-of-the-art performance in locating the outline
of present teeth with a median point-to-curve error of 0.2 mm for each
of the teeth.

**Keywords:** Teeth segmentation · Panoramic dental images
Random forest regression-voting · Machine learning

## 1 Introduction

Dental radiographs have been widely used since the discovery of X-rays in a variety of fields: abnormality detection, treatment and/or surgery planning, prosthe-
ses design, assessment of children's dental development, human identification by
dental matching, and many more. X-ray images provide additional information
to the simple exploration of the oral cavity since they reveal hidden parts of the
teeth and other surrounding structures. There are several types of dental X-ray
images depending on the captured area. In intraoral images, the sensor is placed
inside the mouth and the images cover some specific area (no more than 3–4
complete teeth). In contrast, in extraoral images the sensor is placed outside the
mouth and the images cover a bigger area. That is the case for panoramic images,
which provide a complete coverage of the dentition and other surrounding bones
and tissues with a very small dose of ionising radiation. Although their quality

© Springer Nature Switzerland AG 2019
T. Vrtovec et al. (Eds.): MSKI 2018, LNCS 11404, pp. 11–21, 2019.
https://doi.org/10.1007/978-3-030-11166-3_2

is highly dependent on patient positioning and patient movements during acquisition [1,2] they have been widely used to diagnose periodontal disease, cysts in the jaw bones, jaw tumours, oral cancer, impacted teeth, temporomandibular joint disorders or sinusitis, among others.

One of the key tasks in automatic dental image processing is teeth segmentation. This has proven to be useful in a variety of areas such as human identification [3–5], caries detection [6], lesion detection [7] or even dental age estimation [8]. The works in this area tackled automatic or semiautomatic teeth segmentation mostly from intraoral images in a variety of ways, comprising thresholding [4,9], combination of morphological operations [10,11], active contours [3], level sets [12], mixture of Gaussians [5] and many more. Although these algorithms can reach great performance in a variety of applications, they present some problems when working with dental images, mainly because they are very sensitive to intensity changes, dental restorations, teeth injuries and overlapping teeth. Thus, there is a need to follow more robust approaches which use domain knowledge to improve the results.

In this regard, methods utilising statistical models have proven to be accurate and robust in medical image segmentation. One of latest contributions on this area are random forest regression-voting constrained local models (RFRV-CLMs) [13], which are an evolution of the original constrained local models [14] and combines a global shape model with individual point appearance models. Over the last years, this approach has been applied to a variety of medical images with high performance [15–17], which encourages us to use it in the teeth segmentation problem.

Our main contribution is the development of a fully automatic procedure to outline mandibular adult-stage teeth in panoramic images, including the identification of any missing teeth.

## 2    Methods

### 2.1    RFRV-CLM

RFRV-CLMs combine a linear shape model with a set of local models designed to locate each point. RFRV-CLMs are summarised in the following, and the reader is referred to [13,15] for full details.

Each annotated shape is encoded as a vector $x$ with the concatenated coordinates of the $n$ landmark points; $x = (x_0, y_0, x_1, y_1, \ldots, x_{n-1}, y_{n-1})^T$. In order to train the model, the shapes are resampled and aligned in a reference frame so a linear model can be built as follows:

$$x = T_\theta(\bar{x} + Pb_i + r_i), \tag{1}$$

where $\bar{x}$ is the mean shape, $P$ are eigenvectors of the covariance matrix, $b$ is a vector of shape parameters, $r$ is a regularisation term which allows small deviations from the model and $T_\theta$ is a similarity transformation of parameters $\theta$ which maps the shape from the reference frame to the image frame.

In order to locate each individual point, random forest regression-voting is used. The region of interest which encloses all landmark points is resampled into a standardised reference frame and for each landmark point $l$ in $x$ a set of image patches $p_j$ are sampled at random displacements $d_j$ (i.e. centred at $l+d_j$). Then a set of decision tree regressors are trained from the Haar features [18] of all patches to predict the displacements.

Given a new image and an initial estimation of the pose of the mean shape, the region of interest is resampled into a standardised reference frame and a set of image patches are sampled at random displacements around each initial estimated point. Haar features are extracted from the patches and fed into the random forest regressors. The outputs of all decision trees are accumulated in a voting grid $V_l$, where the positions of the grid with higher values indicate the most likely position for that landmark point.

The local appearance models and the global shape model are combined as follows:

$$Q(b, \theta, r) = \sum_{l=0}^{n-1} V_l(T_\theta(\bar{x}_l + Pb_l + r_l)), \qquad (2)$$

$$\text{s.t.} \quad b^T S_b^{-1} b \le M_t \quad \text{and} \quad |r_l| < r_t,$$

where $M_t$ and $r_t$ are thresholds on the Mahalanobis distance and the regularisation term, respectively, and $S_b$ is the covariance matrix of the shape model parameters $b$. This yields the overall quality-of-fit (QoF) measurement $Q$ (2), which represents the total number of votes for a shape defined by parameters $\{b, \theta, r\}$.

The search process is carried out iteratively, so for each search iteration the algorithm gets the set of parameters $\{b, \theta, r\}$ which maximises the overall QoF and updates the landmark points.

## 2.2  Two-Step Teeth Segmentation

We build separate RFRV-CLMs for each tooth type. Given that the dentition is almost horizontally symmetric, a single model trained from one tooth on one side (left or right) can also be used to segment the corresponding tooth on the opposite side. It is worth mentioning that there are two main problems with teeth segmentation from individual teeth models. First of all, the space occupied by each tooth is very small when compared to the image size, so the search process requires a reasonably good initialisation. Furthermore, teeth of the same type (e.g. single-root and multi-root) are very similar to each other so the search process can easily end up converging to a neighbouring tooth.

To overcome these problems, in addition to individual teeth models, another model was trained from some keypoints in the image. The idea is to identify the most representative points in each tooth and the mandible which give a reasonably good approximation of their poses (see Table 1). Thus, this model is able to capture the pose variation of each tooth (in terms of position, size and rotation) in relation to neighbouring teeth and the mandible. As the mandible occupies a similar percentage in all panoramic images, a good initialisation of the search model can be carried out by placing the mean shape in the centre of the image and scaling it to the 75% of the image width.

The search process for a new image is performed fully automatically in two steps. In the first step, the keypoint model looks for the optimal localisation of the teeth and mandible keypoints. Then, the initial pose estimation of each tooth is carried out via (3):

$$\arg \min_{\theta} d\Big(k_t, T_\theta(\bar{x}_k)\Big), \tag{3}$$

where $k_t$ is the estimation of the keypoints of tooth $t$ provided by the first model, $\bar{x}_k$ are the keypoints of the mean shape of tooth $t$ and $d$ is the Euclidean distance function. The initial shape estimation for each tooth is, therefore, the result of applying the estimated pose to the mean shape, $T_\theta(\bar{x})$.

On completion of the search we estimate the QoF of each model point by computing the magnitude of the mean displacement vector produced by the random forest for the point when evaluated on a patch centred on the point. This should be small for good matches and larger for those points which do not match so well. To obtain a score for the whole tooth we compute the mean, $m$, and standard deviation, $sd$, of the values for each point, and construct the final score as $QoF =, m + sd$. This has been shown to be a more effective discriminator than just using the mean alone. We treat a tooth as missing if this QoF is above a threshold.

## 3    Experiments and Results

In this work, a set of 346 panoramic images provided by the School of Medicine and Dentistry, University of Santiago de Compostela, Spain, have been used, all of which were collected under ethical approval. To test the proposed segmentation approach, the images where one hemi-arch including all seven left-mandibular teeth (from the first incisor to the second molar) were present have been used as the train set, and the remaining images have been used as the test set. In total, 261 images have been used for training and 85 for testing. In each image the shapes of seven left-mandibular teeth (from 31 to 37) have been manually annotated as well as 7 mandible keypoints (see Fig. 1 and Table 1). In total, each training example consists of a set of 263 landmark points.

The individual tooth models and the keypoint model were built using the RFRV-CLM algorithm. The mean shape of each tooth model is shown in Fig. 2. For each model, a coarse-fine approach has been followed, which in this case consists of training a fine model where the reference frame width is approximately the desired object width, and training a coarse model where the frame width is about a quarter of the fine frame width. This gives a rough but more robust shape estimation at first and then refines the shape. In the case of the keypoint model, the search process consists of 3 search iterations with the coarse model

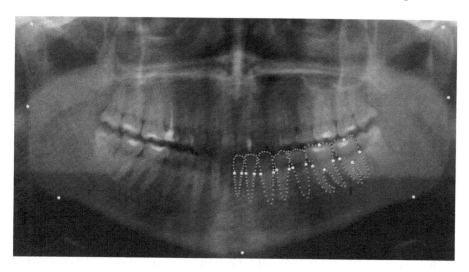

**Fig. 1.** Annotated points in each single image. In red: teeth and mandible keypoints; in blue: teeth non-keypoints. (Color figure online)

and 2 search iterations with the fine model. For the individual teeth models, the iterations of coarse and fine searches have been reduced to 2 and 1, respectively.

The predicted shapes of teeth 31 to 37 have been compared to manually annotated shapes and the performance of the proposed approach has been assessed in three ways. Firstly, the performance of present/missing teeth detection has been measured. Table 2 shows the classification results when choosing a threshold to maximise (true positive rate - false positive rate). See Fig. 4 for some examples. Secondly, to assess whether the have been located correctly, the intersection over union (IoU) of annotated and predicted shapes was calculated from the examples

**Table 1.** Number of points used in each individual model and number of points of each model used in the keypoint model.

| Model | #points | #points used in keypoint model |
|---|---|---|
| Central incisor (31) | 32 | 2 (one on each neck side) |
| Lateral incisor (32) | 32 | 2 (one on each neck side) |
| Canine (33) | 32 | 2 (one on each neck side) |
| First premolar (34) | 32 | 2 (one on each neck side) |
| Second premolar (35) | 32 | 2 (one on each neck side) |
| First molar (36) | 48 | 4 (one on each neck side, one at the top and one at the root bifurcation) |
| Second molar (37) | 48 | 4 (one on each neck side, one at the top and one at the root bifurcation) |
| Mandible | 7 | 7 (nearly equidistant points between the top of the condyles) |

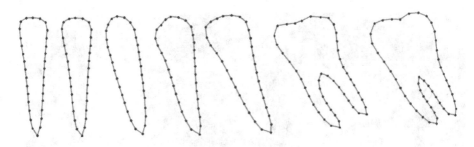

**Fig. 2.** Mean shape of each individual tooth model.

where both teeth are present and are correctly detected as present. Table 3 shows that the detection of multiroot teeth (36 and 37) is slightly more successful than the detection of single root teeth. This is likely to be because the anterior teeth are closer to each other so the model might match a neighbouring tooth. Assuming that an overlap greater than 50% between the prediction and the ground truth indicates that the predicted shape is very likely to match the real tooth, the examples with a IoU value over 0.5 have been treated as correctly located. In general, the proportion of well-located teeth is over 90% among all teeth types. Thirdly, the accuracy of the tooth shape matching has been evaluated on the correctly located teeth (where the overlap between model and true tooth is greater than 50%) with the point-to-curve error, which represents the shortest distance from each estimated point to the curve through the ground truth landmark points (Table 4). The median of the errors is less than 0.23 mm for all types of teeth. The 99%-ile is 1.31 mm in the worst case, which demonstrates the robustness of the proposed segmentation approach. Note that all performance measurements have been obtained on the left mandibular teeth only as we did not have manual ground truth annotations for the right side. However, the right mandibular teeth can be outlined by applying the left mandibular teeth models to the horizontally reflected images. See Fig. 3 for some examples.

**Table 2.** Confusion matrix of the missing teeth detection problem and binary classification metrics. In order to obtain these metrics, the "present" class has been considered as the positive class.

Prediction

| | | Missing | Present | Total | | |
|---|---|---|---|---|---|---|
| | | | | | Accuracy | 95.46% |
| Real | Missing | 31 (TN) | 6 (FP) | 37 | Precision | 98.9% |
| | Present | 21 (FN) | 537 (TP) | 558 | Sensitivity | 96.24% |
| | Total | 53 | 542 | 595 | Specificity | 83.78% |

**Table 3.** Intersection over the union (IoU) statistics for each individual tooth predictions: mean, standard deviation, median. In the last column, the percentage of the examples with an IoU over 0.5, which are treated as correctly located.

| Model | Mean | Sd | Median | % over 0.5 |
|-------|------|------|--------|------------|
| 31 | 0.78 | 0.24 | 0.86 | 89.41% |
| 32 | 0.80 | 0.20 | 0.86 | 92.94% |
| 33 | 0.84 | 0.18 | 0.90 | 94.12% |
| 34 | 0.84 | 0.22 | 0.91 | 91.76% |
| 35 | 0.85 | 0.23 | 0.93 | 92.21% |
| 36 | 0.87 | 0.18 | 0.92 | 95.77% |
| 37 | 0.86 | 0.21 | 0.92 | 94.29% |

## 4    Discussion and Conclusions

We have shown that a state-of-the-art performance can be achieved in adult mandibular teeth segmentation by using the RFRV-CLM algorithm in two steps. The first step provides an estimation of some teeth and mandible keypoints, which are used to initialise each individual tooth search. In the second step, the search of each tooth is performed independently. This two-step approach overcomes the problem of automatically initialising each individual tooth model, and the results show that the teeth shapes can be matched very accurately, especially if the tooth is correctly located.

A limitation of this study is that we have not taken into account the third molar (also known as the *wisdom tooth*). This is because this tooth is often extracted or missing in some patients so we had very few examples. Moreover, although the QoF statistics are a good starting point for missing teeth detection, this task could be improved by using other metrics or algorithms developed specifically for that purpose.

**Table 4.** Point to curve statistics in each individual tooth model (in mm): mean, standard deviation, median and 90, 95 and 99 centiles. These results have been obtained on the examples where the teeth have been correctly located.

| Model | Mean | Sd | Med | 90% | 95% | 99% |
|-------|------|------|------|------|------|------|
| 31 | 0.23 | 0.12 | 0.21 | 0.38 | 0.47 | 0.61 |
| 32 | 0.30 | 0.23 | 0.22 | 0.58 | 0.65 | 1.29 |
| 33 | 0.30 | 0.24 | 0.23 | 0.56 | 0.76 | 1.31 |
| 34 | 0.24 | 0.20 | 0.19 | 0.36 | 0.56 | 0.90 |
| 35 | 0.21 | 0.11 | 0.18 | 0.30 | 0.48 | 0.58 |
| 36 | 0.25 | 0.16 | 0.20 | 0.35 | 0.50 | 0.89 |
| 37 | 0.27 | 0.14 | 0.23 | 0.41 | 0.48 | 0.82 |

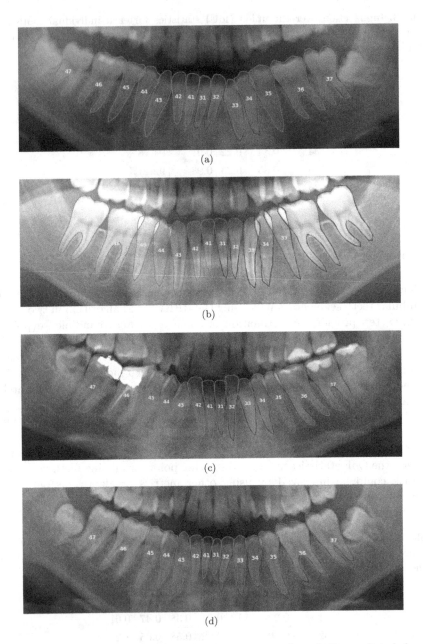

**Fig. 3.** Results of automatic teeth segmentation process. In red, the predicted shapes. In blue, the left-mandibular manually annotated shapes. The segmentation is robust to some issues such as very bright images (b) or tooth filling (c). It also can manage teeth overlapping. It is worth noting that the most noticeable segmentation errors are observed in the apical regions (around root apices) due to the low contrast of the image in that area. (Color figure online)

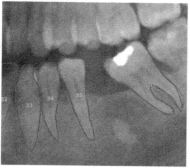
(a) Missing tooth 36 detected correctly.

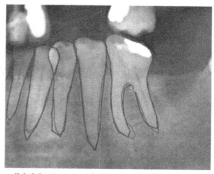
(b) Missing tooth 37 detected correctly.

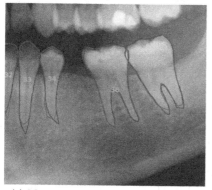
(c) Missing tooth 35 detected correctly.

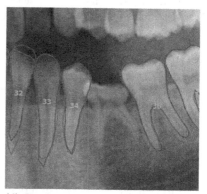
(d) Tooth 35 searcher detects correctly tooth as missing. This is a special clinic case called agenesia, where the tooth (premolar 35 in the image) fails to form, so the related primary tooth is not pushed outward.

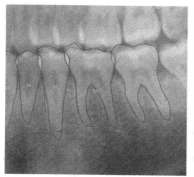
(e) Tooth 37 detected incorrectly as missing.

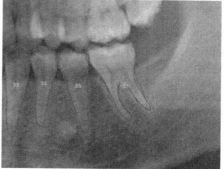
(f) Tooth 37 detected incorrectly as present due to it matches tooth 36.

**Fig. 4.** Results of present/missing teeth detection. In red, the predicted shapes. In blue, the left-mandibular manually annotated shapes. (Color figure online)

Nonetheless, the presented results are promising and are a big step towards a fully automatic dental assessment tool with a variety of applications. Two direct uses of the proposed system are (i) automatic teeth measurements with a view to plan surgical treatments; and (ii) automatic radiograph matching with the aim of identifying people (e.g. in forensics). Other clinical tasks could also be carried out with this system and few functionality additions. For example, the detection of caries, impacted tooth and other abnormalities.

**Acknowledgements.** This work has received financial support from the Consellería de Cultura, Educación e Ordenación Universitaria (accreditation 2016–2019, ED431G/08, growth potential group 2017-2020 ED431B 2017/029, reference competitive group 2017–2020, ED431C 2017/69, and N. Vila Blanco support ED481A-2017) and the European Regional Development Fund (ERDF). C. Lindner is funded by the Medical Research Council, UK (MR/S00405X/1).

# References

1. Rondon, R., Pereira, Y., do Nascimento, G.: Common positioning errors in panoramic radiography: a review. Imaging Sci. Dent. **44**(1), 1–6 (2014). https:// doi.org/10.5624/isd.2014.44.1.1
2. Halperin-Sternfeld, M., Machtei, E., Balkow, C., Horwitz, J.: Patient movement during extraoral radiographic scanning. Oral Radiol. **32**(1), 40–47 (2016). https:// doi.org/10.1007/s11282-015-0208-6
3. Chen, H., Jain, A.: Tooth contour extraction for matching dental radiographs. In: Proceedings of the 17th International Conference on Pattern Recognition – ICPR 2004, vol. 3, pp. 522–525. IEEE (2004). https://doi.org/10.1109/ICPR.2004. 1334581
4. Nomir, O., Abdel-Mottaleb, M.: A system for human identification from X-ray dental radiographs. Pattern Recogn. **38**(8), 1295–1305 (2005). https://doi.org/10. 1016/j.patcog.2004.12.010
5. Chen, H., Jain, A.: Dental biometrics: alignment and matching of dental radiographs. In: Proceedings of the 7th IEEE Workshops on Application of Computer Vision– WACV/MOTION 2005, vol. 1, pp. 316–321. IEEE (2005). https://doi.org/ 10.1109/ACVMOT.2005.41
6. Oliveira, J., Proença, H.: Caries detection in panoramic dental X-ray images. In: Tavares, J., Jorge, R.N. (eds.) Computational Vision and Medical Image Processing. Computational Methods in Applied Sciences, vol. 19, pp. 175–190. Springer, Dordrecht (2011). https://doi.org/10.1007/978-94-007-0011-6_10
7. Li, S., Fevens, T., Krzyżak, A., Jin, C., Li, S.: Semi-automatic computer aided lesion detection in dental X-rays using variational level set. Pattern Recogn. **40**(10), 2861–2873 (2007). https://doi.org/10.1016/j.patcog.2007.01.012
8. Čular, L., Tomaić, M., Subašić, M., Šarić, T., Sajković, V., Vodanović, M.: Dental age estimation from panoramic X-ray images using statistical models. In: Proceedings of the 10th International Symposium on Image and Signal Processing and Analysis – ISPA 2017, pp. 25–30. IEEE (2017). https://doi.org/10.1109/ISPA. 2017.8073563

9. Razali, M., Ahmad, N., Zaki, Z., Ismail, W., et al.: Region of adaptive threshold segmentation between mean, median and Otsu threshold for dental age assessment. In: Proceedings of the International Conference on Computer, Communications, and Control Technology – I4CT 2014, pp. 353–356. IEEE(2014). https://doi.org/10.1109/I4CT.2014.6914204

10. Lira, P., Giraldi, G., Neves, L.: Panoramic dental X-ray image segmentation and feature extraction. In: Proceedings of the V Workshop of Computing Vision, Sao Paulo, Brazil (2009)

11. Amer, Y., Aqel, M.: An efficient segmentation algorithm for panoramic dental images. Procedia Comput. Sci. **65**, 718–725 (2015). https://doi.org/10.1016/j.procs.2015.09.016

12. Shah, S., Abaza, A., Ross, A., Ammar, H.: Automatic tooth segmentation using active contour without edges. In: Proceedings of the 2006 Biometrics Symposium: Special Session on Research at the Biometric Consortium Conference, pp. 1–6. IEEE(2006). https://doi.org/10.1109/BCC.2006.4341636

13. Lindner, C., Bromiley, P., Ionita, M., Cootes, T.: Robust and accurate shape model matching using random forest regression-voting. IEEE Trans. Pattern Anal. Mach. Intell. **37**(9), 1862–1874 (2015). https://doi.org/10.1109/TPAMI.2014.2382106

14. Cristinacce, D., Cootes, T.: Automatic feature localisation with constrained local models. Pattern Recognit. **41**(10), 3054–3067 (2008). https://doi.org/10.1016/j.patcog.2008.01.024

15. Lindner, C., Thiagarajah, S., Wilkinson, J., Wallis, G., The arcOGEN Consortium: Fully automatic segmentation of the proximal femur using random forest regression voting. IEEE Trans. Med. Imaging **32**(8), 1462–1472 (2013). https://doi.org/10.1109/TMI.2013.2258030

16. Cootes, T.F., Ionita, M.C., Lindner, C., Sauer, P.: Robust and accurate shape model fitting using random forest regression voting. In: Fitzgibbon, A., Lazebnik, S., Perona, P., Sato, Y., Schmid, C. (eds.) ECCV 2012. LNCS, vol. 7578, pp. 278–291. Springer, Heidelberg (2012). https://doi.org/10.1007/978-3-642-33786-4_21

17. Bromiley, P.A., Adams, J.E., Cootes, T.F.: Localisation of vertebrae on DXA images using constrained local models with random forest regression voting. In: Yao, J., Glocker, B., Klinder, T., Li, S. (eds.) Recent Advances in Computational Methods and Clinical Applications for Spine Imaging. LNCVB, vol. 20. Springer, Cham (2015). https://doi.org/10.1007/978-3-319-14148-0_14

18. Viola, P., Jones, M.: Rapid object detection using a boosted cascade of simple features. In: Proceedings of the 2001 IEEE Conference on Computer Vision and Pattern Recognition – CVPR 2001. IEEE (2001). https://doi.org/10.1109/CVPR.2001.990517

# Fully Automatic Planning of Total Shoulder Arthroplasty Without Segmentation: A Deep Learning Based Approach

Paul Kulyk[1,2], Lazaros Vlachopoulos[3], Philipp Fürnstahl[3], and Guoyan Zheng[1(✉)]

[1] Institute for Surgical Technology and Biomechanics, University of Bern, Bern, Switzerland
guoyan.zheng@istb.unibe.ch
[2] College of Medicine, University of Saskatchewan, Saskatoon, Canada
[3] Computer Assisted Research and Development Group, University of Zurich, Balgrist University Hospital, Zurich, Switzerland

**Abstract.** We present a method for automatically determining the position and orientation of the articular marginal plane (AMP) of the proximal humerus in computed tomography (CT) images without segmentation or hand-crafted features. The process is broken down into 3 stages. Stage 1 determines a coarse estimation of the AMP center by sampling patches over the entire image and combining predictions with a novel kernel density estimation method. Stage 2 utilizes the estimate from stage 1 to focus on a smaller sampling region and operates at a higher images resolution to obtain a refined prediction of the AMP center. Stage 3 focuses patch sampling on the region around the center obtained at stage 2 and regresses the tip of a vector normal to the AMP which yields the orientation of the plane. The system was trained and evaluated on 27 upper arm CTs. In a 4-fold cross-validation the mean error in estimating the AMP center was $1.30 \pm 0.65$ mm and the angular error for estimating the normal vector was $4.68 \pm 2.84°$.

**Keywords:** Regression · Proximal humerus
Articular marginal plane · Deep learning · Total shoulder arthroplasty

## 1 Introduction

Shoulder arthroplasty is a common orthopaedic procedure indicated in certain cases of primary and secondary degenerative conditions. The annual rate of shoulder arthroplasty has been increasing with a steeper increase in total shoulder arthroplasty (TSA) compared to hemiarthroplasty since the early 2000s. In 2008, an estimated 46,951 procedures were performed in the USA (20,178 hemiarthroplasties and 26,773 total shoulder arthroplasties) [1]. Both of these

T. Vrtovec et al. (Eds.): MSKI 2018, LNCS 11404, pp. 22–34, 2019.
https://doi.org/10.1007/978-3-030-11166-3_3

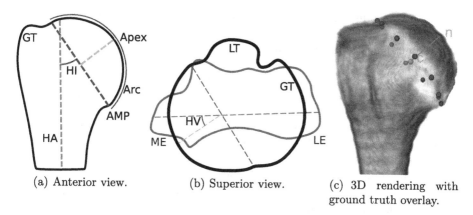

(a) Anterior view.        (b) Superior view.        (c) 3D rendering with ground truth overlay.

**Fig. 1.** Key dimensions of the proximal humerus: GT = greater tuberosity, HA = humeral axis, HI = humeral head inclination, HV = humeral head version, LE = lateral epicondyle, LT = lesser tuberosity, ME = medial epicondyle. Figure (c) shows the hand-selected points defining the articular marginal plane in blue as well as the calculated ground truth center and normal in green. (Color figure online)

procedures require replacing the humeral joint surface with TSA addressing the glenoid surface as well. This paper focuses on determining the location and orientation of the humeral head.

Preservation of articular anatomy with the purpose of maintaining physiologic soft tissue tension is the motivation behind humeral implant design. Traditional long-stemmed monobloc humeral implants have, for the most part, been replaced by modular versions and more recently short-stemmed, stemless, or resurfacing implants have gained popularity [2]. These modern implants allow adjustments that can fit the implant to match the anatomy encountered intra-operatively. They typically rely on resection of the humeral head along the anatomic neck, which is approximated geometrically by the articular marginal plane (AMP). In many cases this resection is done freehand intraoperatively; however, recognition of the importance of accurately reconstructing the humeral head anatomically is becoming more relevant, particular with short-stemmed, stemless, and resurfacing implants [2–4].

**Table 1.** Normal dimensions of the humeral head.

| Parameter | Mean | Normal range |
|---|---|---|
| Radius of curvature | 22 to 25 mm | 17 to 32 mm |
| Articular surface arc | 150° | Not provided |
| Thickness | 15 to 20 mm | 12 to 24 mm |
| Inclination | 40 to 45° | 30 to 55° |
| Version | $-18$ to $-25°$ | 5 to $-60°$ |

A high variability exists in the anatomy of the proximal humerus, typical accepted mean values summarized by Keener et al. [2] are shown in Fig. 1 and Table 1. Our focus will be defining where the center of the AMP is and its orientation in space. Further work would be required to define the humeral axis and epicondylar axis, from which the inclination and version could be defined. This provides motivation for today's modular systems which can be adapted to a wide range of anatomical variations.

With modular systems, often a detailed preoperative analysis of the anatomic dimensions is not performed except in cases of extreme deformity or small size where special order or patient-specific components may be required. Simple templating using X-rays and scaled two-dimensional (2D) drawings of implants to visually confirm restoration of anatomy is often all that is performed preoperatively [3]. The surgeon can adjust the exact orientation and size components intraoperatively and determine appropriate fit by soft tissue assessment. The importance of the exact level of accuracy of the humeral component parameters is not well defined; however, it is suggested that restoration of the physiologic anatomy and forces would provide most success in restoring the kinematics of the shoulder and reducing shear stresses on the glenoid component [2,5]. Accurate measurement of the AMP will likely become more important in cases such as resurfacing and stemless implants where the implant positioning is based directly off of the AMP.

Most implant companies provide surgeons with planning software that allows overlay of implant models on three-dimensional (3D) computed tomography (CT) data. Manual positioning of the virtual components can allow the surgeon to determine the appropriate size and position of components preoperatively, as well as to determine reaming and cutting trajectories. The information from these systems can currently also be used to produce patient specific guides that improve reproducibility of glenoid instrumentation guide pins [3].

Previous work has defined the AMP by manually selecting points on the anatomic neck on CT data and producing a best-fit plane to this [6,7]. This is time consuming and its accuracy is prone to inter-observer variations [8]. Recently, Tschannen et al. [9] sought to automate the process using a random forest-based method. They compared their method to a manually-assisted atlas-based method and were able to improve accuracy.

Automated regression of landmarks using deep learning methods has seen recent success in several applications [10–12]. Automatic and computer-assisted techniques for determination of the glenoid parameters have been investigated and shown success in providing accurate information for preoperative planning [13–15]. The humeral head remains relatively neglected, with Tschannen et al. [9] being the only study identified regarding automatic parameter recovery. An attempt to create a system to improve the accuracy of automatic determination of the AMP utilizing fully convolutional neural networks will be explored. Our method will rely on a CT scan cropped roughly such that it must include the humeral head and from this predict the location and orientation of the AMP automatically.

# 2    Materials and Methods

## 2.1    Method Overview

The aim of the project is to develop a deep learning-based method to automatically determine the AMP given an upper arm CT scan without segmentation or hand-crafted features. To fully define the AMP we require a point in the plane and a vector normal to it giving the orientation. We propose a 3-stage, multiscale, cascaded system to achieve this. Each stage samples patches from the image and predicts an offset from the patch location to the desired landmark. The results are combined to form a prediction for the landmark at each stage. The first stage processes patches from the CT volume at a low resolution and combines them to predict a rough estimate for the center of the AMP. The second stage refines the center estimate by running at a higher resolution and focusing training at a region of interest (ROI) centered at the stage 1 prediction. Finally, the third stage runs at the higher resolution to predict the tip of the normal vector thus giving all the information required to define the AMP.

## 2.2    Data Description

We used 27 cropped CT scans of *right* shoulders from the previous work of Tschannen et al. [9]. The data were collected from the Institutes for Forensic Medicine of the Universities of Bern and Zurich, Switzerland. The CT scanners used were a Siemens Emotion 6® and a Siemens Somaton Definition Flash®. The cropped images typically had a field of view $228.6 \times 228.6 \times 450$ mm (covering the area used clinically for assessing the upper arm) and a typical resolution of $1.27 \times 1.27 \times 0.6$ mm though there were some scans that varied slightly from these parameters. All images were resampled into a isometric low and high resolution voxel size of $1.25 \times 1.25 \times 1.25$ mm and $0.6 \times 0.6 \times 0.6$ mm respectively.

The AMP was defined by 12 manually picked points[1] along the margin where articular cartilage transitions to bone. From these points our regression targets, the AMP center and the tip of the normal vector, were derived. The original 12 points were shifted to have a mean at the origin. Using singular value decomposition we obtained the orientation of this plane, yielding the normal. Performing least-squares fitting to a circle of the points projected into this plane defines the AMP center. The center and normal vector were then shifted back to the original location using the original mean.To define a single point for the patch-based regression, the tip of the normal vector was defined as the point where a normal emanating from the center of the AMP intersected the surface of the humeral head. The ground truth points overlaid on a 3D view of the proximal humerus are shown in Fig. 1(c).

## 2.3    Network Architecture

Inspired by the landmark regression FCN introduced in our previous work [10], here we designed patch-based FCNs to solve our problem. More specifically,

---

[1] Performed by an expert in the Tschannen et al. [9] group.

we opted to utilize a multiscale approach with the regression split into three stages, each stage processes multiple patches in prediction mode and uses a modified kernel density estimation (KDE) to combine the information into a single prediction. The architecture defining our system is shown in Fig. 2.

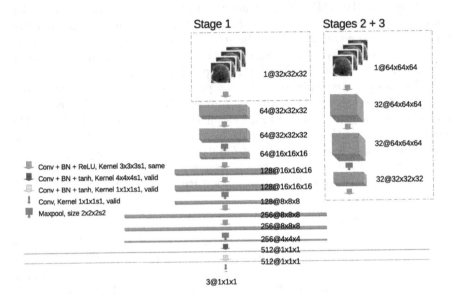

**Fig. 2.** The network used is shown with the output being the offset from the patch corner to the center of the articular marginal plane. Layer dimensions given in the form: `channels @ patch shape`. Stages 2 and 3 use the same layout but add an additional repeat of the convolution/convolution/maxpool structure to match the dimensions.

**Stage 1.** This low resolution stage utilizes an input patch size of $32 \times 32 \times 32$ voxels at a voxel size of $1.25 \times 1.25 \times 1.25$ mm. It generates a rough estimate of the AMP center location, which allows for a refinement at stage 2. It begins with a scheme repeated three times consisting of two 3D convolutions (each with a kernel of $3 \times 3 \times 3$, a stride of 1, batch normalization, and a rectified linear unit, ReLU, activation) followed by max pooling (with size $2 \times 2 \times 2$ and a stride of 2). Next a convolution with kernel $4 \times 4 \times 4$, stride 1, batch normalization, and an hyperbolic tangent (tanh) as activation[2] reduces the patch dimensions to $1 \times 1 \times 1$. Another convolution with kernel $1 \times 1 \times 1$, stride 1, batch normalization, and a tanh activation reduces the patch dimensions to $1 \times 1 \times 1$. Finally, a convolution with kernel $1 \times 1 \times 1$, stride 1, no batch normalization, and no activation[3] reduces the patch dimensions to 3 values representing the three coordinates of the displacement from the patch location to the target landmark.

---

[2] When tested during development tanh produced a better loss than ReLU when used in these stages. Possibly due to the fact that tanh does not force the output to positive numbers.

[3] Foregoing the activation function allows this stage to produce the full range of floats as possible outputs.

**Stages 2 and 3.** These higher resolution stages utilize the same network structure as stage 1 with the exception that they take as input a patch size of $64 \times 64 \times 64$ voxels at a voxel size of $0.6 \times 0.6 \times 0.6$ mm in order to produce a regression with higher accuracy. To divide the larger patch size to the same output there are 4 repetitions of the input stages instead of 3. Stage 3 utilizes the same network definition as stage 2; however, it is trained to regress the tip of the normal vector instead of the center of the AMP.

## 2.4   Training

Previous work has suggested that limiting patch selection to points on edges has the potential to improve training time and accuracy [10,16]. We adopted this by generating Canny edge maps for each image, sampling patches only from the voxels located on edges. Additionally, the region nearer to the humeral head is likely to have more relevant information on its pose [9], so we designed a new sampling strategy to sample more points in regions nearer to the humeral head as described below.

During training all patches were obtained from a spherical region of radius $r_{max}$ separated into shells of equal width, $r_{shell}$, centered at the ground truth center of the AMP as illustrated in Fig. 3. Each batch consisted of a number of samples, $n_s$, from a single image divided equally among the shells so that more patches were sampled from regions nearer to the center. The parameters for sampling for each stage are listed in Table 2.

**Table 2.** Sampling parameters (ROI: region of interest).

| Stage | Batch size $n_s$ | ROI radius $r_{max}$ (voxels) | Shell width $r_{shell}$ (voxels) |
|-------|------------------|-------------------------------|----------------------------------|
| 1 | 128 | 64 | 16 |
| 2 | 32 | 64 | 16 |
| 3 | 32 | 32 | 16 |

During each epoch, each image was visited once in a newly randomized order and a different random sampling of patches was obtained. The mean-squared error loss function was used representing the Euclidean distance between predicted displacement and the ground truth displacement. The Adam optimizer algorithm with an exponential decay of the learning rate was employed [17]. Each stage is trained independently.

## 2.5   Testing

Testing proceeds in a cascaded fashion as shown in Fig. 4. Given an unseeen CT volume, stage 1 samples patches uniformly over the entire volume and generates

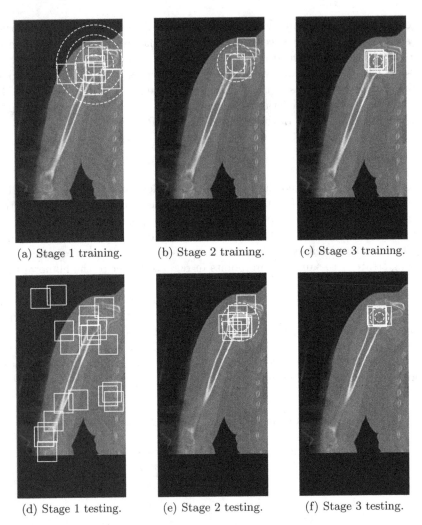

(a) Stage 1 training.    (b) Stage 2 training.    (c) Stage 3 training.

(d) Stage 1 testing.    (e) Stage 2 testing.    (f) Stage 3 testing.

**Fig. 3.** During training an equal number of patches are sampled from each spherical shell centered at the ground truth center with a smaller region of interest in each subsequent stage. During testing stage 1 samples randomly from the entire volume and generates a rough center prediction, $c_1$. Stage 2 prediction uses shells centered at $c_1$ to predict $c_2$ which is used in turn as the center for the sampling shells in stage 3.

a prediction at the lower resolution for the center of the AMP. This prediction is used as a center for the spherical sampling ROI in stage 2, concentrating the higher resolution patches at the region around the humeral head. From stage 2 we obtain a more accurate estimate of the AMP center which we also use as the ROI center for stage 3 sampling. Stage 3 finally produces a prediction for the normal vector tip. Sampling is illustrated in Fig. 3 and the parameters used are in Table 2.

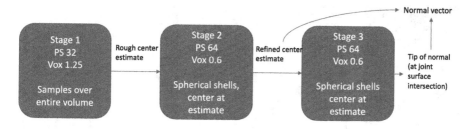

**Fig. 4.** Pipeline of predictions using the 3-stage network.

At each stage 1024 patches are sampled and processed to generate a single prediction. The network returns a 3D offset vector to the predicted landmark location for each processed patch. Each patch in the sample set has a known location and thus generates an independent prediction for the location of the landmark. To improve the accuracy, the independent predictions are combined using an approximate KDE to generate a 3D probability map as described below.

**Fast KDE Implementation.** Typical KDE implementations are computationally intensive, a novel algorithm was implemented to generate a probability map by only calculating the kernel to 2 standard deviations along each direction. The standard deviation for each direction was approximated from the covariance in the distribution of landmark locations from the prediction sample set. This clipped Gaussian kernel was added to a 3D array of zeros the same size as the image centered at each prediction location generating a non-normalized approximate probability distribution. The location of the maximum value in this array was taken as the prediction of the landmark. The typical appearance of a prediction at each stage is shown in Fig. 5.

## 2.6   Implementation Details

The network described was trained and tested using Tensorflow 1.5 [18] in Python 3.6.5 on a Tesla 1080 Ti GPU using an Ubuntu Linux 16.04 workstation with an Intel Core i7-7700 CPU at 3.60 GHz and 32 GB RAM.

## 2.7   Experimental Design

We evaluated the accuracy of the present approach using a standard 4-fold cross-validation experiment. To this end, the set of 27 images provided was split into 3 groups of 7 images and 1 group of 6. For every fold of study, 3 out of 4 groups of data were used for training and the left-out group were used for testing. Stage 1 and 2 were trained 500 epochs and stage 3 was trained 100 epochs. The accuracy was evaluated by comparing the prediction for each of the images as described in Sect. 2.5 to the corresponding ground truth.

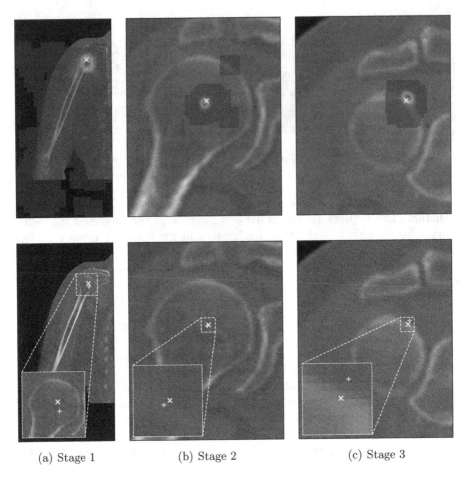

(a) Stage 1          (b) Stage 2          (c) Stage 3

**Fig. 5.** Example of predictions shown in the $xz$-plane through the ground truth location. The first row shows a typical kernel density estimation heatmap, the second shows the ground truth position ($\times$) and the predicted location ($+$).

The error in the center of the AMP and vector tip predictions are defined as an L2 distance from the prediction to the associate ground truth. The angular error is determined by solving the cosine relationship for the angle between the predicted normal and the ground truth $\theta$:

$$\theta = \arccos \left( \frac{\mathbf{u} \cdot \mathbf{v}}{|\mathbf{u}| \cdot |\mathbf{v}|} \right). \tag{1}$$

## 3   Results

The mean error for estimating the center of the AMP is $1.30 \pm 0.65$ mm. The mean angular error was $4.68 \pm 2.84°$. A scatter plot showing the distribution for each prediction grouped by fold is shown in Fig. 6. Figures 6 and 7 demonstrate the distribution of our error measurements for the center of the AMP, the vector tip, and the angular error, respectively. In order to compare the estimation uncertainty of different quantities, we calculated the coefficient of variations $(CV)$ for each quantity. We found $CV_{center} = 50\%$, $CV_{vector} = 42.1\%$, and $CV_{angular} = 60.7\%$, respectively, suggesting higher uncertainty in our angular error results. The uncertainty in estimating the normal vector is increased by the fact that we are compounding the error of the location of both the AMP center and the normal tip (calculated by 2 separate networks) when we compute the normal vector (Table 3).

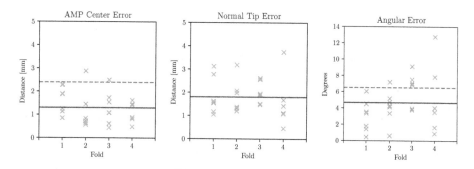

**Fig. 6.** Error shown for each prediction in the dataset, grouped by validation fold. Mean displayed as a blue line, mean of random forest-based method shown as a green dashed line for comparison. (Color figure online)

**Table 3.** Mean error of each validation fold.

| Fold | Center error (mm) | Vector tip error (mm) | Angular error ($°$) |
|------|-------------------|-----------------------|---------------------|
| 1 | $1.66 \pm 0.54$ | $1.84 \pm 0.74$ | $3.01 \pm 1.79$ |
| 2 | $1.12 \pm 0.77$ | $1.76 \pm 0.67$ | $4.21 \pm 1.84$ |
| 3 | $1.28 \pm 0.65$ | $1.99 \pm 0.42$ | $6.45 \pm 1.79$ |
| 4 | $1.12 \pm 0.41$ | $1.58 \pm 1.04$ | $5.1 \pm 4.08$ |
| All | $1.30 \pm 0.65$ | $1.78 \pm 0.75$ | $4.68 \pm 2.84$ |
| [9] | $2.4 \pm 1.2$ | Not applicable | $6.51 \pm 3.43$ |

## 4    Discussion

Accurate location and orientation of the AMP are key to planning the resection of the humeral head in both TSA and hemiarthroplasty. The level of accuracy needed in final humeral head orientation for a successful outcome is not fully defined; however, it is certainly an important factor in preserving the anatomical orientation of the proximal humerus which is key to successful kinematics

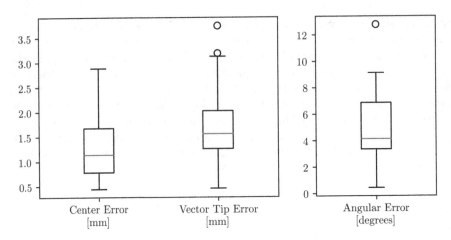

**Fig. 7.** Distribution of error in predictions.

and glenoid loading [2,5]. Modern modular humeral implants as well as short-stemmed, stemless, and resurfacing techniques are focus attention on anatomical replacement of the humeral head [2]. To date, more work has been directed toward computer-assisted planning methods for the glenoid component. The only automated method for determining the parameters of AMP identified was Tschannen et al. [9].

Our results of a mean error for the center of the AMP of $1.30 \pm 0.65$ mm and a mean angular error of $4.68 \pm 2.84°$ are an improvement on the prior work. Additionally, our choice to restrict the ROI to an area around the humeral head in training seems to have supported Tschannen et al. [9] in assuming this is the area containing the most relevant information for determining the parameters of the AMP.

The data from this technique also yields the height of the humeral head directly as the length of the normal vector, though this was not assessed for accuracy at this time. Additional information, such as the radius of the AMP, could be regressed with the given ground truth information simply by regressing an additional point in a similar fashion to stage 3. With this information one could fully define the parameters of humeral head. An additional system could be developed to define the orientation of the humeral shaft, combined with our approach this could fully define the humeral implant parameters as per Fig. 1. Our work could be integrated into computer-assisted surgery systems to provide a cutting plan for resection of the AMP. Deep learning methods offer an extendible, highly accurate method of regressing parameters from medical imaging data that does not rely on hand-selected features. They may be more readily extended to new applications than traditional machine learning techniques.

# References

1. Kim, S., Wise, B., Zhang, Y., Szabo, R.: Increasing incidence of shoulder arthroplasty in the United States. J. Bone Joint Surg. Am. **93**(24), 2249–2254 (2011). https://doi.org/10.2106/JBJS.J.01994
2. Keener, J., Chalmers, P., Yamaguchi, K.: The humeral implant in shoulder arthroplasty. J. Am. Acad. Orthop. Surg. **25**(6), 427–438 (2017). https://doi.org/10.5435/JAAOS-D-15-00682
3. Edwards, T., Morris, B., Gartsman, G.: Shoulder Arthroplasty, 2nd edn. Elsevier, Amsterdam (2019)
4. Dines, D., Laurencin, C., Williams, G. (eds.): Arthritis & Arthroplasty: The Shoulder. Saunders/Elsevier, Philadelphia (2009)
5. Pearl, M.: Proximal humeral anatomy in shoulder arthroplasty: implications for prosthetic design and surgical technique. J. Shoulder Elbow Surg. **14**(Suppl 1), S99–S104 (2005). https://doi.org/10.1016/j.jse.2004.09.025
6. DeLude, J., et al.: An anthropometric study of the bilateral anatomy of the humerus. J. Shoulder Elbow Surg. **16**(4), 477–483 (2007). https://doi.org/10.1016/j.jse.2006.09.016
7. Johnson, J., Thostenson, J., Suva, L., Hasan, S.: Relationship of bicipital groove rotation with humeral head retroversion: a three-dimensional computed tomographic analysis. J. Bone Joint Surg. Am. **95**(8), 719–724 (2013). https://doi.org/10.2106/JBJS.J.00085
8. Vlachopoulos, L., et al.: Computer algorithms for three-dimensional measurement of humeral anatomy: analysis of 140 paired humeri. J. Shoulder Elbow Surg. **25**(2), e38–e48 (2016). https://doi.org/10.1016/j.jse.2015.07.027
9. Tschannen, M., Vlachopoulos, L., Gerber, C., Székely, G., Fürnstahl, P.: Regression forest-based automatic estimation of the articular margin plane for shoulder prosthesis planning. Med. Image Anal. **31**, 88–97 (2016). https://doi.org/10.1016/j.media.2016.02.008
10. Janssens, R., Zeng, G., Zheng, G.: Fully automatic segmentation of lumbar vertebrae from CT images using cascaded 3D fully convolutional networks. arXiv:1712.01509 (2017).
11. Payer, C., Štern, D., Bischof, H., Urschler, M.: Regressing heatmaps for multiple landmark localization using CNNs. In: Ourselin, S., Joskowicz, L., Sabuncu, M.R., Unal, G., Wells, W. (eds.) MICCAI 2016. LNCS, vol. 9901, pp. 230–238. Springer, Cham (2016). https://doi.org/10.1007/978-3-319-46723-8_27
12. Zhang, J., et al.: Joint craniomaxillofacial bone segmentation and landmark digitization by context-guided fully convolutional networks. In: Descoteaux, M., Maier-Hein, L., Franz, A., Jannin, P., Collins, D., Duchesne, S. (eds.) MICCAI 2017. LNCS, vol. 10434, pp. 720–728. Springer, Cham (2017). https://doi.org/10.1007/978-3-319-66185-8_81
13. Boileau, P., Cheval, D., Gauci, M., Holzer, N., Chaoui, J., Walch, G.: Automated three-dimensional measurement of glenoid version and inclination in arthritic shoulders. J. Bone Joint Surg. Am. **100**(1), 57–65 (2018). https://doi.org/10.2106/JBJS.16.01122
14. Nguyen, D., et al.: Improved accuracy of computer assisted glenoid implantation in total shoulder arthroplasty: an in-vitro randomized controlled trial. J. Shoulder Elbow Surg. **18**(6), 907–914 (2009). https://doi.org/10.1016/j.jse.2009.02.022

15. Werner, B., Hudek, R., Burkhart, K., Gohlke, F.: The influence of three-dimensional planning on decision-making in total shoulder arthroplasty. J. Shoulder Elbow Surg. **26**(8), 1477–1483 (2017). https://doi.org/10.1016/j.jse.2017.01.006

16. Suzani, A., Seitel, A., Liu, Y., Fels, S., Rohling, R.N., Abolmaesumi, P.: Fast automatic vertebrae detection and localization in pathological CT scans - a deep learning approach. In: Navab, N., Hornegger, J., Wells, W.M., Frangi, A.F. (eds.) MICCAI 2015. LNCS, vol. 9351, pp. 678–686. Springer, Cham (2015). https://doi.org/10.1007/978-3-319-24574-4_81

17. Kingma, D., Ba, J.: Adam: a method for stochastic optimization. arXiv:1412.6980 (2014)

18. Abadi, M., et al.: TensorFlow: a system for large-scale machine learning. arXiv:1605.08695 (2016)

# Deep Volumetric Shape Learning for Semantic Segmentation of the Hip Joint from 3D MR Images

Guodong Zeng and Guoyan Zheng[✉]

Institute for Surgical Technology and Biomechanics, University of Bern,
Bern, Switzerland
guoyan.zheng@istb.unibe.ch

**Abstract.** This paper addresses the problem of segmentation of the hip joint including both the acetabulum and the proximal femur in three-dimensional magnetic resonance images. We propose a fully convolutional volumetric auto encoder that learns a volumetric representation from manual segmentation in order to regularize the segmentation results obtained from a fully convolutional network. We further introduce a super resolution network to improve the segmentation accuracy. Comprehensive results obtained from 24 patient data demonstrated the effectiveness of the proposed framework.

**Keywords:** Deep learning · Hip joint · Semantic segmentation
Shape learning · Super resolution

## 1 Introduction

Femoroacetabular impingement (FAI) is a cause of hip pain in adults and has been recognized recently as one of the key risk factors that may lead to the development of early cartilage and labral damage [1] and a possible precursor of hip osteoarthritis [2]. Several studies [2,3] have shown that the prevalence of FAI in young populations with hip complaints is high. Although there exist a number of imaging modalities that can be used to diagnose and assess FAI, magnetic resonance (MR) imaging does not induce any dosage of radiation at all and is regarded as the standard tool for FAI diagnosis [4]. While manual analysis of a series of two-dimensional (2D) MR images is feasible, automated segmentation of the proximal femur in MR images will greatly facilitate the applications of MR images for FAI surgical planning and simulation.

The topic of automated MR image segmentation of the hip joint has been addressed by a few studies which relied on atlas-based segmentation [5], graph-cut [6], active models [7,8] or statistical shape models [9]. While these methods reported encouraging results for bone segmentation, further improvements are needed. For example, Arezoomand et al. [8] recently developed a three-dimensional (3D) active model framework for segmentation of the proximal femur in MR images and they reported an average recall of 0.88.

© Springer Nature Switzerland AG 2019
T. Vrtovec et al. (Eds.): MSKI 2018, LNCS 11404, pp. 35–48, 2019.
https://doi.org/10.1007/978-3-030-11166-3_4

Recently, machine-learning based methods, especially those based on convolutional neural networks (CNNs), have witnessed successful applications in natural image processing [10,11] as well as in medical image analysis [12–15]. For example, Prasoon et al. [12] developed a method to use a triplanar CNN that can autonomously learn features from images for knee cartilage segmentation. More recently, 3D volume-to-volume segmentation networks were introduced, including 3D U-Net [13], 3D V-Net [14] and a 3D deeply supervised network [15].

In this paper, we propose a fully convolutional volumetric auto-encoder that learns a volumetric latent representation from manual segmentation in order to regularize the segmentation results obtained from a fully convolutional network (FCN). To derive the volumetric latent representation from such a fully convolutional volumetric auto-encoder and to further use the derived latent representation to regularize segmentation are memory intensive as both steps require to take volumes containing the complete structures as input. To address such a difficulty, we propose to conduct the latent space constrained segmentation in a downsampling space and then introduce a super resolution network to improve the segmentation resolution, leading to improved segmentation accuracy. The details about our method will be presented in Sect. 2. We will then describe the experiments and results in Sect. 3, followed by a discussion in Sect. 4.

## 2    Method

Figure 1 illustrates the proposed method for hip joint segmentation. It contains three networks, i.e. a FCN-based segmentation network, a denoising autoencoder and a super resolution network. Our method takes a down-sampled low resolution (LR) MR image as input and directly generate high resolution (HR) segmentation. Below we first present an overview of the proposed method, followed by the presentation of the loss functions, network architectures, and the implementation details.

### 2.1    Overview

The FCN-based segmentation network is to segment the input low resolution MR image $x_l$ into 3 classes, i.e. acetabulum, femur and background. The denoising autoencoder is to learn a latent representation from manual volumetric segmentation in order to regularize the output from the FCN-based segmentation network.

The low resolution MR image and the segmentation from the denoising autoencoder provide complementary information: the low resolution MR image provides original density information, while the segmentation from the denoising autoencoder provides the anatomically constrained segmentation probabilities. The super resolution network takes both the low resolution MR image and the anatomically constrained segmentation from the denoising autoencoder as input to generate the final segmentation in high resolution.

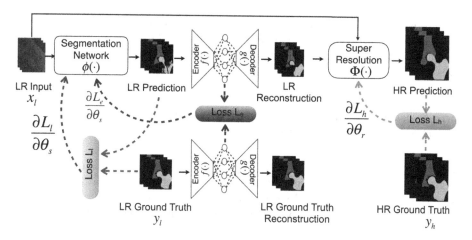

**Fig. 1.** A schematic view of the proposed method for the hip joint segmentation.

## 2.2   Loss Functions

We train our network in three stages: in the first stage, the segmentation network (Snet) and autoencoder (AE) were trained separately. Then the segmentation network was trained jointly with the autoencoder. In the third stage, the super resolution network was trained to upscale the output of the decoder to a high resolution segmentation.

Before we introduce the details of loss functions, we need to do some definitions. The input MR image in high resolution (HR) and low resolution (LR) are defined as $x_h$ and $x_l$, respectively. The segmentation ground truth in HR and LR are defined as $y_h$ and $y_l$, respectively. The function $f(\cdot)$ and $g(\cdot)$ are defined as the encoder and decoder components of the AE, respectively. $\phi(\cdot)$ and $\Phi(\cdot)$ are defined as the segmentation network and super resolution network, respectively.

**Loss Function of Snet and AE at Stage One.** Snet is to segment the low resolution input MR Images $x_l$ into several sub-classes, including acetabulum, femur and background. AE is to learn a latent representation so that the segmentation input can be reconstructed. Specifically, the training objective of AE is shown below:

$$\min_{\theta_e} \{L_{mce}(g(f(y_l)), y_l) + \lambda_w \|w_e\|_2^2 \}, \tag{1}$$

where $\theta_e$ denotes all trainable parameters of the AE model and $w_e$ denotes all trainable parameters except bias term in the AE network, $\lambda_w$ determines the weight of decay terms, and $L_{mce}$ a multi-class cross entropy loss ($mce$) defined as:

$$L_{mce} = -\frac{1}{N} \sum_{i=1}^{N} \sum_{c=1}^{C} y_{ic} \log \hat{y_{ic}}, \tag{2}$$

where $N$ is the number of samples, $C$ is the number of classes, $\hat{y}_{ic}$ is the predicted probability and $y_{ic}$ is the corresponding ground truth label.

For the segmentation network trained in the first stage, which aims to minimizes a voxel-wise multi-class cross entropy loss, i.e. $L_l$, which is shown below:

$$L_l(x_l, y_l; \theta_s) = L_{mce}(\phi(x_l), y_l) + \lambda_w \|w_s\|_2^2, \tag{3}$$

where $\theta_s$ denotes all trainable parameters of Snet and $w_s$ denotes all trainable parameters except bias term in Snet.

**Loss Function of Snet at Stage Two.** In stage two, the AE network was integrated into the segmentation network. The segmentation network was trained not only to minimize the voxel-wise cross-entropy loss, but also to minimize the Euclidean loss $L_e$ of the latent representation learnt by AE. $L_e$ is defined as below:

$$L_e(x_l, y_l) = \|f(\phi(x_l)) - f(y_l)\|_2^2, \tag{4}$$

The training of the segmentation network in the second stage is shown as follows:

$$\min_{\theta_s} \{L_{mce}(\phi(x_l), y_l) + \lambda_1 L_e + \lambda_w \|w_s\|_2^2 \}. \tag{5}$$

**Loss Function of Snet at Stage Three.** In the third stage, the super resolution network was trained to upscale the low resolution segmentation, i.e. the output of decoder in AE, to high resolution segmentation. The loss of the super resolution network is defined as below:

$$L_h(x_l, y_h; \theta_r) = L_{mce}(\Phi(g(f(\phi(x_l)))), y_h) + \lambda_w \|w_r\|_2^2, \tag{6}$$

where $\theta_r$ denotes all trainable parameters of the super resolution network and $w_r$ denotes all trainable parameters except bias term in the super resolution network.

### 2.3 Network Architectures

Below we present the network architectures of different sub-networks involved in our method.

**Segmentation Network.** Figure 2 illustrates the architecture of the segmentation network. It is a variant of the 3D U-net [13].

**Denoising Autoencoder.** Figure 3 shows the architecture of the fully convolutional denoising auto encoder to learn an end-to-end, voxel-to-voxel mapping. The left half of our network can be seen as an encoder stage that results in a condensed representation (indicated by "latent vector representation"). In the second stage (right half), the network reconstructs back the input from the latent vector representation by deconvolutional (3DDeconv) layers. The network is trained using cross-entropy loss. After training, the encoder $f(y; \theta_f)$ can be used to map a noisy volumetric label to a vector representation $h$ in the latent space.

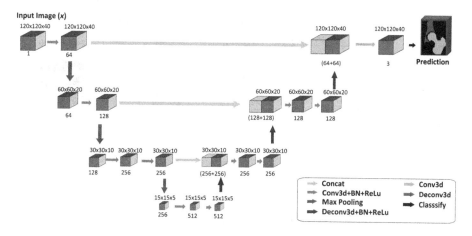

**Fig. 2.** The architecture of the segmentation network.

**Super Resolution Network.** Figure 4 illustrates the architecture of super resolution network. The input of the super resolution network is the concatenation of the low resolution MR image and the segmentation probability map reconstructed from the denoising autoencoder. After one convolutional layer to the input, the feature maps were upscaled by $2 \times 2 \times 2$ times through a deconvolutional layer. Followed by another two convolutional layers, the segmentation in high resolution was generated.

All convolutional and deconvolutional layers are followed by a BN layer [16] and a ReLU layer [17], except the last one before the final output layer. All filter size of convolutional and deconvolutional layers are $3 \times 3 \times 3$.

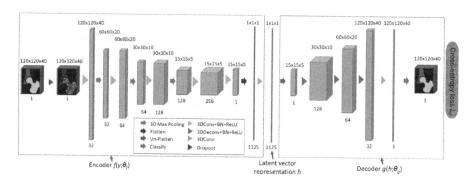

**Fig. 3.** The architecture of the fully convolutional denoising autoencoder for volumetric representation.

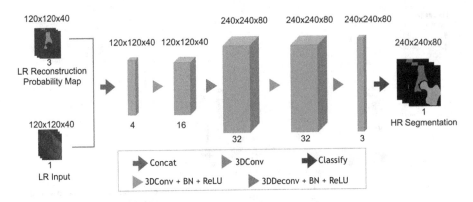

**Fig. 4.** The architecture of super resolution network.

### 2.4   Implementation Details

The proposed method was implemented in Python using TensorFlow framework on a desktop with a 3.6 GHz Intel(R) i7 CPU and a GTX 1080 Ti graphics card with 11 GB GPU memory.

**Training.** The whole volume of MR images in low resolution are fed into the neural network, and the size is $120 \times 120 \times 40$. Each training volumetric image was normalized as zero mean and unit variance. As we train our three networks (segmentation network, autoencoder, and super resolution network) in an end-to-end way, the batch size of 1 was adopted. We trained our networks from scratch, and all weights were initialized from a Gaussian distribution ($\mu = 0, \sigma = 0.01$). As mentioned above, the training was done in three stages. The segmentation network and autoencoder were trained separately for 10,000 iterations, and all weights were updated by the stochastic gradient descent (SGD) algorithm (momentum $= 0.9$, weight decay $= 0.005$). After that, we started the second stage training, i.e. the segmentation network and autoencoder were jointly trained for another 10000 iterations. In the final stage, the super resolution network was trained for another 10000 iterations. In total, we trained our neural network for 30000 iterations. For each stage of the training, the initial learning rate was $1 \times 10^{-3}$ and halved by 3000 every training iterations.

**Testing.** In the inference phase, the high resolution MR image was downscaled to a low resolution MR image in the size of $120 \times 120 \times 40$, and the trained model can directly generate the high resolution segmentation results.

## 3   Experiments and Results

We conduct a series experiments: First we evaluate the reconstruction performance of the trained denoising autoencoder model. Then we compared different methods on the hip joint segmentation. Metrics used to evaluate the performance include the Dice overlap coefficient (Dice) [18], Hausdorff distance (HD) [19], average surface distance (ASD) [20], and precision and recall [21].

### 3.1 Dataset and Preprocessing

The dataset contains 24 hip joint data of FAI patients. All data are in the format of volumetric MR images and in the size of $240 \times 240 \times 80$ (high resolution). To feed the whole volume data into the neural network, all MR images were downscaled to $120 \times 120 \times 40$ (low resolution). Further, to enlarge the training samples and mitigate possible over-fitting problem, random noise was injected: random value between $(-3, 3)$ was added to each voxel. Finally, each training sample was normalized as zero mean and unit variance before being fed into the network.

### 3.2 Denoising Autoencoder Experiments

In this experiment, we conduct experiments to evaluate the performance of the denoising autoencoder in terms of shape completion and false positive exclusion. Standard two-fold cross validation were adopted. The dataset was randomly split into two separate parts, 12 were used for training and 12 were used for testing.

The qualitative results from the denoising autoencoder are shown in Fig. 5. The top half of the figure illustrates the shape completion function of the denoising autoencoder. Specifically, the input labels are randomly dropped by 50% percent and become incomplete-shaped labels with lots of "holes". And the denoising autoencoder generates labels without holes but with complete shape. The bottom half of the figure shows the false positive exclusion function of denoising autoencoder. The input labels are added with 50% random noise and become noisy input with lots of false positive predictions. Again the denoising autoencoder generates labels with complete shape and almost no false positive predictions.

We further explore how much shape corruption and noise that the denoising autoencoder can tolerate. Specifically, we are going to find the minimum percentage of original labels that the model needed and the maximum percentage of noise that the model can tolerate when it can still make accurate reconstruction. Table 1 shows the quantitative results about the relationship between the dropout rate of the input labels and the reconstruction accuracy. We can observe that even with a dropout rate of 95%, i.e. only 5% of the original labels are kept, the model can still make good reconstruction. But when the dropout rate was increased to 99%, ASD of both acetabulum and femur are larger than 1 mm, which is assumed as a bad reconstruction.

Based on the maximum dropout rate (95%), we explore the maximum noise level that the model can tolerate. Table 2 shows the quantitative results about the relationship between the noise level and the reconstruction accuracy. As one can observe from the results, even with 75% of random noise, the denoising autoencoder can still make good reconstruction. When the noise level is

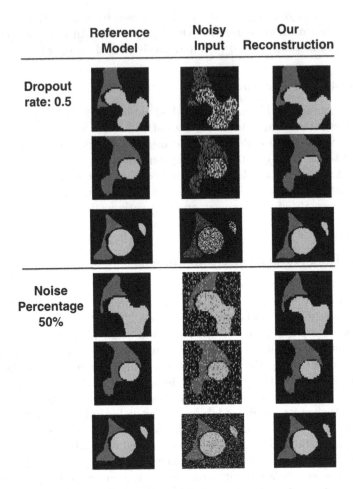

**Fig. 5.** Shape reconstruction with dropout and random noise.

**Table 1.** Dropout rate and reconstruction accuracy (Dice: Dice overlap coefficient; ASD: average surface distance).

| Dropout rate | Acetabulum | | Femur | |
|---|---|---|---|---|
| | Dice | ASD (mm) | Dice | ASD (mm) |
| 0.50 | 0.928 | 0.42 | 0.957 | 0.37 |
| 0.75 | 0.925 | 0.44 | 0.955 | 0.40 |
| 0.90 | 0.913 | 0.54 | 0.947 | 0.47 |
| 0.95 | 0.894 | 0.67 | 0.936 | 0.64 |
| 0.99 | 0.810 | **1.45** | 0.892 | **1.06** |

**Table 2.** Noise level and reconstruction accuracy (Dice: Dice overlap coefficient; ASD: average surface distance).

| Noise level (%) | Acetabulum | | Femur | |
|---|---|---|---|---|
| | Dice | ASD (mm) | Dice | ASD (mm) |
| 25 | 0.885 | 0.75 | 0.931 | 0.65 |
| 35 | 0.876 | 0.80 | 0.932 | 0.66 |
| 50 | 0.873 | 0.83 | 0.930 | 0.66 |
| 75 | 0.856 | 0.96 | 0.922 | 0.74 |
| 100 | 0.842 | **1.07** | 0.921 | 0.78 |

increased to 100%, the average ASD of acetabulum is increased to 1.07 mm and the reconstruction is corrupted.

Based on above analysis, we would say the trained denoising autoencoder model can make good reconstructions with only 5% of original input labels and have a tolerance of 75% noise. Figure 6 shows an example of reconstruction with both corruption labels and noise.

The results demonstrate that the model can reconstruct hip shapes based on little image information and with high noise tolerance. This raises the question of whether it simply represents a fixed shape. Figure 7 shows four reconstructions randomly selected from the 12 test cases. Even though the shapes of the acetabulum vary considerably, the model fits each image accurately, demonstrating that it models the full range of acetabular shapes represented in the input data.

### 3.3 Segmentation Experiments

In this experiment, the proposed method is applied to segment the hip joint from 3D MR images using the dataset described in Sect. 3.1. We conduct a standard two-fold cross validation to evaluate the performance.

The proposed method is compared with: patch-based 3DUnet [13] model in high resolution (HR-3DUnet), whole-volume based 3DUnet model in low res-

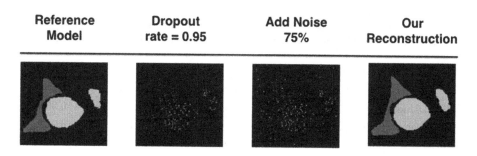

**Fig. 6.** Shape reconstruction with dropout and random noise.

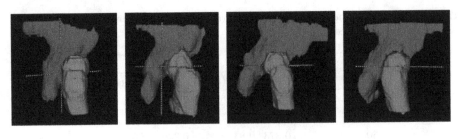

**Fig. 7.** Randomly selected shape reconstruction examples.

olution (LR-3DUnet) and the cascaded 3DUnet with AE model regularization (AE-Seg) [22]. The experiment results are shown in Table 3.

From the experiments results shown in Table 3, we can observe HR-3DUnet significantly under-performs compared with other methods in terms of Dice (0.842 for acetabulum and 0.873 for femur), HD (65.91 mm for acetabulum and 40.67 mm for femur) and ASD (7.80 mm for acetabulum and 6.49 mm for femur). The poor performance is also shown in the qualitative comparison in Fig. 8. The segmentation results from HR-3DUnet contains many more false positive detections compared with LR-3DUnet, especially in the axial view and sagittal view. This is due to the fact that HR-3DUnet adopts a patch-based strategy, and a patch cannot take advantage of the global context information. But global context information is critically important in the task of hip joint segmentation, because the gray value of acetabulum, femur and background are very similar, and the boundary is also very fuzzy.

LR-3DUnet takes the whole low resolution volume as input, encouraging the segmentation results to make more use of global context. All evaluation metrics shown in Table 3 from LR-3DUnet are better than HR-3DUnet. But LR-3DUnet suffer from the voxel-wise loss, which cannot guarantee the global consistency and meaningful structure. For the segmentation results from LR-3DUnet, the mean ASD of acetabulum and femur are 1.79 mm and 1.60 mm, respectively, which are quite large compared to good segmentations. In addition, there are many false positives predictions, especially in the coronal view, which can be seen in the third line of Fig. 8.

**Table 3.** Quantitative comparison of segmentation results (Dice: Dice overlap coefficient; HD: Hausdorff distance; ASD: average surface distance; Prec.: precision).

| Methods | Acetabulum | | | | | Femur | | | | |
|---|---|---|---|---|---|---|---|---|---|---|
| | Dice | HD | ASD | Prec. | Recall | Dice | HD | ASD | Prec. | Recall |
| HR-3DUnet | 0.842 | 65.91 | 7.80 | 0.754 | 0.961 | 0.873 | 40.67 | 6.49 | 0.804 | 0.965 |
| LR-3DUnet | 0.860 | 24.76 | 1.79 | 0.813 | 0.916 | 0.893 | 14.60 | 1.60 | 0.865 | 0.927 |
| AE-Seg | 0.885 | 29.23 | 1.17 | 0.884 | 0.890 | 0.907 | 11.62 | 0.84 | 0.926 | 0.896 |
| Ours | 0.899 | 20.19 | 0.67 | 0.912 | 0.888 | 0.933 | 9.29 | 0.58 | 0.942 | 0.926 |

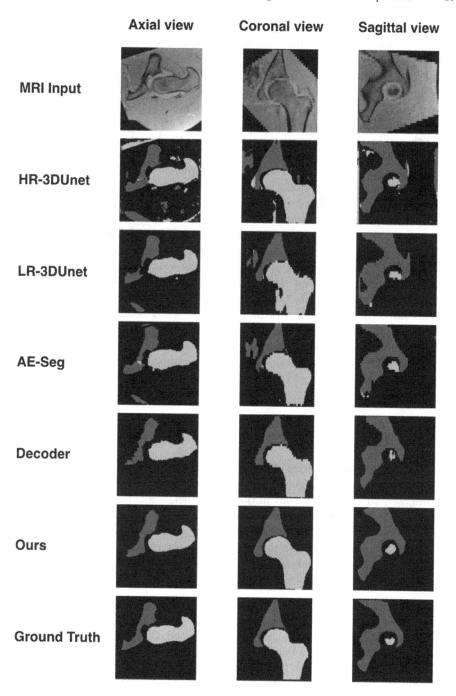

**Fig. 8.** Comparison of segmentations from different methods.

AE-Seg [22] makes use of an implicit way to constrain the segmentation shape and implements it as a regularization term in the training phase. However, it is too weak to force the network to generate segmentations that completely lie in the latent space. In the fourth row of Fig. 8, we can see that AE-Seg can partially remove some false positives in the sagittal view, but the false positive predictions in the axial view and the coronal view still cannot be eliminated. For the acetabulum of a hip joint, its shape is complex and has large differences from each other. This is due to regularization term on the latent representation works in an implicit way and cannot really guarantee segmentation with meaningful shape. That is also why though there is an improvement in Dice for acetabulum, compared with LR-3DUnet, the average HD metric (29.23 mm) from AE-Seg is even worse than LR-3DUnet (24.76 mm).

Our method explicitly constrains the segmentation shape via the denoising autoencoder. The outputs from the denoising autoencoder were shown in the fifth row of Fig. 8. The denoising autoencoder can automatically remove false positives and fill some missing parts by prior knowledge.

The comparison between the segmentation results by our method and the ground truth is shown in last two bottom lines in Fig. 8. This comparison clearly demonstrates the effectiveness of incorporating the denoising autoencoder and super resolution network to generate final segmentation results. The quantitative comparison in Table 3 also demonstrated the efficacy of the proposed method. Compared with HR-3DUnet, our method has an improvement of 5.7% and 6.0% over HR-3DUnet in terms of Dice for segmenting the acetabulum and the proximal femur, respectively.

## 4   Discussion

Incorporating prior knowledge into image segmentation algorithms has proven useful in order to obtain more accurate and plausible results [23]. In this paper, we proposed to use a fully convolutional volumetric auto encoder to learn volumetric representation in order to regularize the segmentation output of a segmentation network. We further introduced a super resolution network to improve the segmentation accuracy. We conducted comprehensive experiments on 3D MR images of 24 patients to validate the efficacy of the proposed method.

## References

1. Laborie, L., Lehmann, T., Engesæter, I., Eastwood, D., Engesæter, L., Rosendahl, K.: Prevalence of radiographic findings thought to be associated with femoroacetabular impingement in a population-based cohort of 2081 healthy young adults. Radiology **260**(2), 494–502 (2011). https://doi.org/10.1148/radiol.11102354
2. Leunig, M., Beaulé, P., Ganz, R.: The concept of femoroacetabular impingement: current status and future perspectives. Clin. Orthop. Relat. Res. **467**(3), 616–622 (2009). https://doi.org/10.1007/s11999-008-0646-0

3. Clohisy, J., Knaus, E., Hunt, D., Lesher, J., Harris-Hayes, M., Prather, H.: Clinical presentation of patients with symptomatic anterior hip impingement. Clin. Orthop. Relat. Res. **467**(3), 638–644 (2009). https://doi.org/10.1007/s11999-008-0680-y
4. Perdikakis, E., Karachalios, T., Katonis, P., Karantanas, A.: Comparison of MR-arthrography and MDCT-arthrography for detection of labral and articular cartilage hip pathology. Skeletal Radiol. **40**(11), 1441–1447 (2011). https://doi.org/10.1007/s00256-011-1111-9
5. Xia, Y., Fripp, J., Chandra, S., Schwarz, R., Engstrom, C., Crozier, S.: Automated bone segmentation from large field of view 3D MR images of the hip joint. Phys. Med. Biol. **58**(20), 7375–7390 (2013). https://doi.org/10.1088/0031-9155/58/20/7375
6. Xia, Y., Chandra, S., Engstrom, C., Strudwick, M., Crozier, S., Fripp, J.: Automatic hip cartilage segmentation from 3D MR images using arc-weighted graph searching. Phys. Med. Biol. **59**(23), 7245–7266 (2014). https://doi.org/10.1088/0031-9155/59/23/7245
7. Gilles, B., Magnenat-Thalmann, N.: Musculoskeletal MRI segmentation using multi-resolution simplex meshes with medial representations. Med. Image Anal. **14**(3), 291–302 (2010). https://doi.org/10.1016/j.media.2010.01.006
8. Arezoomand, S., Lee, W., Rakhra, K., Beaulé, P.: A 3D active model framework for segmentation of proximal femur in MR images. Int. J. Comput. Assist. Radiol. Surg. **10**(1), 55–66 (2015). https://doi.org/10.1007/s11548-014-1125-6
9. Chandra, S., Xia, Y., Engstrom, C., Crozier, S., Schwarz, R., Fripp, J.: Focused shape models for hip joint segmentation in 3D magnetic resonance images. Med. Image Anal. **18**(3), 567–578 (2014). https://doi.org/10.1016/j.media.2014.02.002
10. Krizhevsky, A., Sutskever, I., Hinton, G.: ImageNet classification with deep convolutional neural networks. In: Pereira, F., et al. (eds.) Proceedings of Neural Information Processing Systems – NIPS 2012, vol. 25, pp. 1097–1105. NIPS (2012)
11. Long, J., Shelhamer, E., Darrell, T.: Fully convolutional networks for semantic segmentation. In: Proceedings of IEEE Conference on Computer Vision and Pattern Recognition – CVPR 2015, pp. 3431–3440. IEEE (2015). https://doi.org/10.1109/CVPR.2015.7298965
12. Prasoon, A., Petersen, K., Igel, C., Lauze, F., Dam, E., Nielsen, M.: Deep feature learning for knee cartilage segmentation using a triplanar convolutional neural network. In: Mori, K., Sakuma, I., Sato, Y., Barillot, C., Navab, N. (eds.) MICCAI 2013. LNCS, vol. 8150, pp. 246–253. Springer, Heidelberg (2013). https://doi.org/10.1007/978-3-642-40763-5_31
13. Çiçek, Ö., Abdulkadir, A., Lienkamp, S.S., Brox, T., Ronneberger, O.: 3D U-net: learning dense volumetric segmentation from sparse annotation. In: Ourselin, S., Joskowicz, L., Sabuncu, M.R., Unal, G., Wells, W. (eds.) MICCAI 2016. LNCS, vol. 9901, pp. 424–432. Springer, Cham (2016). https://doi.org/10.1007/978-3-319-46723-8_49
14. Milletari, F., Navab, N., Ahmadi, S.A.: V-Net: fully convolutional neural networks for volumetric medical image segmentation. In: Proceedings of 4th International Conference on 3D Vision – 3DV 2016, pp. 565–571. IEEE (2016). https://doi.org/10.1109/3DV.2016.79
15. Dou, Q., et al.: 3D deeply supervised network for automated segmentation of volumetric medical images. Med. Image Anal. **41**, 40–54 (2017). https://doi.org/10.1016/j.media.2017.05.001
16. Ioffe, S., Szegedy, C.: Batch normalization: accelerating deep network training by reducing internal covariate shift. In: Proceedings of 32nd International Conference on Machine Learning – ICML 2015, vol. 37, pp. 448–456. PLMR (2015)

17. Dahl, G., Sainath, T., Hinton, G.: Improving deep neural networks for LVCSR using rectified linear units and dropout. In: Proceedings of IEEE International Conference on Acoustics, Speech and Signal Processing – ICASSP 2013, pp. 8609–8613. IEEE (2013). https://doi.org/10.1109/ICASSP.2013.6639346

18. Karasawa, K., et al.: Multi-atlas pancreas segmentation: atlas selection based on vessel structure. Med. Image Anal. **39**, 18–28 (2017). https://doi.org/10.1016/j.media.2017.03.006

19. Huttenlocher, D., Klanderman, G., Rucklidge, W.: Comparing images using the Hausdorff distance. IEEE Trans. Pattern Anal. Mach. Intell. **15**(9), 850–863 (1993). https://doi.org/10.1109/34.232073

20. Yeghiazaryan, V., Voiculescu, I.: An overview of current evaluation methods used in medical image segmentation. Technical report CS-RR-15-08, University of Oxford, Department of Computer Science, UK (2015)

21. Davis, J., Goadrich, M.: The relationship between precision-recall and ROC curves. In: Proceedings of 23rd International Conference on Machine Learning – ICML 2006, pp. 233–240. ACM (2006). https://doi.org/10.1145/1143844.1143874

22. Ravishankar, H., Venkataramani, R., Thiruvenkadam, S., Sudhakar, P., Vaidya, V.: Learning and incorporating shape models for semantic segmentation. In: Descoteaux, M., Maier-Hein, L., Franz, A., Jannin, P., Collins, D.L., Duchesne, S. (eds.) MICCAI 2017. LNCS, vol. 10433, pp. 203–211. Springer, Cham (2017). https://doi.org/10.1007/978-3-319-66182-7_24

23. Nosrati, M., Hamarneh, G.: Incorporating prior knowledge in medical image segmentation: a survey. arXiv:1607.01092 (2016). https://arxiv.org/abs/1607.01092

# Pelvis Segmentation Using Multi-pass U-Net and Iterative Shape Estimation

Chunliang Wang[1(✉)], Bryan Connolly[2], Pedro Filipe de Oliveira Lopes[3],
Alejandro F. Frangi[3], and Örjan Smedby[1]

[1] Department of Biomedical Engineering and Health Systems,
KTH Royal Institute of Technology, Stockholm, Sweden
`chunwan@kth.se`
[2] Radiology Department, Karolinska Institute, Solna, Sweden
[3] Center for Computational Imaging and Simulation Technologies in Biomedicine,
The University of Sheffield, Sheffield, UK

**Abstract.** In this report, an automatic method for segmentation of the pelvis in three-dimensional (3D) computed tomography (CT) images is proposed. The method is based on a 3D U-net which has as input the 3D CT image and estimated volumetric shape models of the targeted structures and which returns the probability maps of each structure. During training, the 3D U-net is initially trained using blank shape context inputs to generate the segmentation masks, i.e. relying only on the image channel of the input. The preliminary segmentation results are used to estimate a new shape model, which is then fed to the same network again, with the input images. With the additional shape context information, the U-net is trained again to generate better segmentation results. During the testing phase, the input image is fed through the same 3D U-net multiple times, first with blank shape context channels and then with iteratively re-estimated shape models. Preliminary results show that the proposed multi-pass U-net with iterative shape estimation outperforms both 2D and 3D conventional U-nets without the shape model.

**Keywords:** Deep learning · Multi-pass U-net · Pelvis segmentation
Shape context · Statistic shape model

## 1 Introduction

Improving resolution of computed tomography (CT) scanners and recent advances in three-dimensional (3D) printing technology make image-guided custom treatment planning and custom implant design more feasible than ever before. However, the timely creation of accurate models of a patient's anatomical structures from 3D high-resolution medical images remains a non-negligible challenge. This challenge limits the clinical applicability of new personalised image-based approaches. As a crucial step in surgery planning, radiotherapy

© Springer Nature Switzerland AG 2019
T. Vrtovec et al. (Eds.): MSKI 2018, LNCS 11404, pp. 49–57, 2019.
https://doi.org/10.1007/978-3-030-11166-3_5

planning and quantitative disease evaluation, pelvis segmentation is often done manually in clinical practice. It can take half an hour to several hours for a trained radiologist to segment the complete pelvis, which is not acceptable in most public hospitals [1].

Several automated and semi-automated segmentation methods have been developed to address this problem. The methods range from intensity thresholding-based approaches, to clustering-based approaches and deformable-model-based approaches [1–4]. However, most existing methods have achieved moderate success only on a few cases. In this study, we tried to evaluate a new deep-learning-based pelvis segmentation method on a relatively large dataset of 90 patients. In recent years, deep-learning-based methods have gained more and more attention due to their superior performance in several image segmentation challenges [5,6]. The deep neural networks are often trained on a large number of training samples in a more or less black-box manner. The neural network learns task-specific image features and rules by minimizing the objective function often correlated with the segmentation error. However, these learned features and rules are difficult to interpret. One can only imagine that the classification decision is based on local appearance and global shapes represented by a stack of convolution kernels and mixed through weighted non-linear rules. The consensus from existing literature is that shape prior knowledge is crucial for accurate and robust pelvis segmentation [1]. The most promising conventional pelvis segmentation methods are based on either statistical shape models or multi-atlas registration [1,3,7]. How to enforce shape prior in a deep learning framework and whether that helps to improve segmentation performance remains an open question. In a previous study [8], Wang et al. proposed a method where statistical shape models were combined with 2.5D U-net to segment multiple structures of the heart in 3D MRI and CT images. In their setup, three two-dimensional (2D) U-nets were first trained to segment the multiple heart structures in three orthogonal views, and then the probability maps were combined and used to estimate 3D shape models of the heart and ventricles. The estimated shapes combined with input images are fed to a second set of 2D U-nets to deliver a refined segmentation result. In this study, a similar strategy was adopted and 3D U-net was trained to take both the 3D CT image and estimated volumetric shape models of the targeted structures as input to generate the segmentation results. However, instead of training two U-nets, the same 3D U-net was retrained multiple times, first with blank images as shape context channels, and then with volumetric shape representation estimated on the preliminary segmentation results. During the testing phase, the input image was passed through the trained 3D U-net several times, with iteratively re-estimated shape context information. In the preliminary experiments performed, the proposed method delivered better segmentation results than the conventional methods using 2D or 3D U-net or statistical shape model methods.

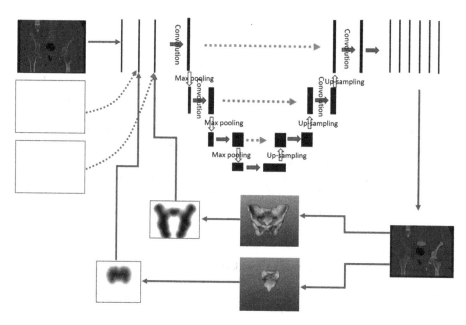

**Fig. 1.** Overview of the proposed multi-pass three-dimensional U-net with iterative shape model estimation.

## 2   Methods

The proposed framework consists of a multi-pass 3D U-net with iterative shape model estimation as summarized in Fig. 1. The core module of this framework is a 3D U-net that takes 3 channels as input: one containing the 3D CT image, two other with the shape context images. The network outputs 6 probability maps for the background, left femur, right femur, left hip bone, right hip bone and sacrum, respectively. The U-net architecture was initially proposed by Ronneberger et al. [6]. In this study we simply extend it to process 3D images instead of 2D images. The 3D U-net consists of 3 max pooling layers and 3 up-sampling layers, and two convolutional layers with kernel size of $3 \times 3 \times 3$ located between max pooling or/and up-sampling layers. Due to limited GPU memory, the input volume size to the U-net is set to $128 \times 128 \times 72$. Original CT data are down-sampled to 3 mm isotropic resolution before being split into overlapping 3D patches of required size. The outputs of the U-net are passed on to a level-set-based volumetric statistical shape estimation module where the shapes of the whole pelvis (including hip bones and sacrum as a whole) and the sacrum bone are estimated. The volumetric shape images are then added to the corresponding input channels and trigger the 3D U-net to re-run. The segmentation and shape estimation loop can be repeated several times until no significant changes occur.

## 2.1  Data Set and Ground Truth Generation

For this work 90 abdominal and pelvis CT scans were selected from public databases (50 from the CT Colonography study [9], 40 from the Lymph Nodes study [10]). Imaging protocols for these studies are available at [9] and [10] respectively. The scans selected were checked to guarantee full coverage of the pelvis, i.e. all pelvic bones are contained in the scan without being partially cut off. Ground-truth segmentation masks were created by an experienced radiologist, using an interactive segmentation tool based on fuzzy connectedness and the level set method. Besides the interactive segmentation, all segmentation masks were carefully inspected and manually edited by the radiologist using the manual segmentation tool in ITKSnap 3.6.0 [11]. On average, each case took between 30 to 50 m to complete the interactive segmentation and manual mask curation procedure.

## 2.2  Statistical Shape Model Creation

The so-called shape context, or shape image, is a volumetric representation of the subject's shape, which is a signed distance map from the surface of the segmented object. However, instead of performing distance transform on the segmentation result directly, a statistical shape model is fit to it to eliminate irregularity that may present in the segmentation results. A statistical model is created by averaging of the signed distance maps of several segmented subjects (training subjects) and computing the main variations using principal component analysis (PCA) [12]. In this study, the shape model is created using 20 randomly selected training subjects, in which the top 10 principal components are computed via PCA. As suggested by Leventon et al., the shape model $M$ that matches the current segmentation is estimated by solving a level set function

$$\frac{\partial \phi}{\partial t} = \alpha F(x) + \beta M(T(x)) + \gamma \kappa(x) |\nabla \phi|, \qquad (1)$$

where $F$ is the image force related to the probability output by the U-net, $M$ is the statistical model as a weighted sum of the mean shape and modes of variation, $T$ is the global transformation and $\kappa$ is the mean curvature. The transformation $T$ and the weighting factors of modes of variation are updated iteratively by minimizing the squared distance between the model and the level set function, which is also a signed distance map. $\alpha$, $\beta$ and $\gamma$ are weighting factors that can be determined empirically.

## 2.3  Training Phase

In the proposed framework, the statistical shape model training is performed only once, but the multi-pass 3D U-net must be trained in two steps. The first step is to train the net by feeding the 3D CT volumes and blank shape context volumes (all voxels are set to zero) to the 3D U-net, which will force the network

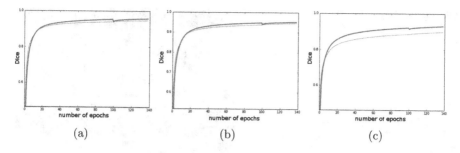

**Fig. 2.** Dice coefficient of (a) the right femur, (b) right hip bone and (c) sacrum bone during the two-step training (first step: 0 – 100 epochs, second step: 100 – 140 epochs). Thick line: training set. Thin line: testing set.

to learn the segmentation using only CT images. In the second step, the pre-trained U-net is retrained with the 3D CT volumes and the real shape context volumes generated from fitting the statistical shape models to the output of the pre-trained 3D U-net. As the weights of the network were already initialized to recognize anatomical structures from the CT channel, the U-net is expected to learn gradually to use the context information where it helps to improve the segmentation results, instead of heavily relying on the context layer. For the U-net training, categorical cross entropy was used as the loss function, stochastic gradient descent as optimizer and the learning rate was set to 0.01. The network was first trained for 100 epochs in the first-step training and 40 epochs in the second-step training (Fig. 2). Sample augmentation was used, where random translating, rotating and scaling are added when creating the training images.

### 2.4    Testing Phase

During testing, the input images were first sent to the trained 3D U-net with blank shape context layers, and then patient-specific shape models were created by fitting the statistical shape model to the preliminary segmentation results. The shape models were added as context layers to the 3D U-net to re-generate the segmentations. The process can be repeated several times. Besides image resampling and intensity normalization, no pre-processing steps are required for the proposed multi-pass U-net segmentation.

## 3    Results

To test the performance of the proposed method, a 5-fold cross validation was performed using the 90 cases. In each fold, 72 subjects were used for training and 18 subjects were used for testing. Both the 3D U-net and the statistical shape models are retrained in every fold. For comparison, the hierarchical statistical shape model based segmentation method reported in [13] was implemented. Plain 2D and 3D U-nets were also trained on the same dataset and compared with

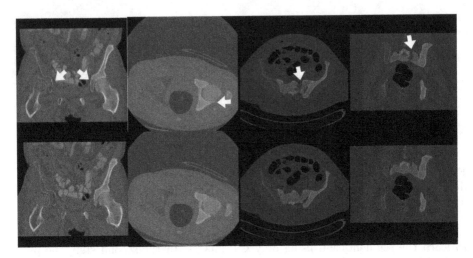

**Fig. 3.** Comparison of results from the first-pass segmentation (top row) and the second-pass segmentation (bottom row). Arrows indicate examples of segmentation errors.

the proposed method. The average segmentation accuracy of 5 bone structures of the pelvis from the 90 subjects is summarized in Table 1. On average, running a 2-pass 3D U-net delivers better results than a 3D U-net. The performance gain is more visible on the sacrum than on other bone structures. Figure 3 shows several examples where adding the shape context component helped to improve the segmentation results. Running the multi-pass U-net for the third time will slightly improve the segmentation accuracy, but no significant improvement is observed when run over 3 iterations. For each fold, the training took 60 h on a NVIDIA GTX 1080ti GPU. For testing, the U-net prediction takes 20–30 s to process a 3D volume, and the shape model estimation takes 2–3 m for each pass.

**Table 1.** Segmentation accuracy measured as dice coefficient of the proposed method and alternative methods.

| Methods | Statistical shape model | 2D U-net axial view | 3D U-net | 1st-pass 3D U-net with blank context | 2nd-pass 3D U-net with shape context | 3rd-pass 3D U-net with shape context |
|---------|------------------------|---------------------|----------|-------------------------------------|-------------------------------------|-------------------------------------|
| Left femur | - | $0.925 \pm 0.178$ | $0.949 \pm 0.039$ | $0.937 \pm 0.047$ | $0.958 \pm 0.032$ | $0.958 \pm 0.031$ |
| Right femur | - | $0.939 \pm 0.122$ | $0.953 \pm 0.019$ | $0.942 \pm 0.026$ | $0.961 \pm 0.018$ | $0.962 \pm 0.018$ |
| Left hip | $0.915 \pm 0.065$ | $0.940 \pm 0.079$ | $0.947 \pm 0.016$ | $0.947 \pm 0.020$ | $0.957 \pm 0.012$ | $0.958 \pm 0.013$ |
| Right hip | $0.908 \pm 0.059$ | $0.943 \pm 0.054$ | $0.947 \pm 0.016$ | $0.944 \pm 0.021$ | $0.957 \pm 0.011$ | $0.957 \pm 0.011$ |
| Sacrum | $0.850 \pm 0.082$ | $0.894 \pm 0.056$ | $0.905 \pm 0.032$ | $0.909 \pm 0.029$ | $0.921 \pm 0.028$ | $0.924 \pm 0.027$ |

# 4  Discussion and Conclusion

The main contribution of the proposed method is to explicitly integrate shape information into a 3D deep neural network, while previously shape context has only been tested in 2D neural networks. The results suggest that adding shape context information to a deep neural network seems to improve the segmentation accuracy, especially for relatively challenging anatomical structures like the sacrum. Our previous paper [8] reported similar findings when adding shape context to 2D U-net. Moving to 3D U-net is important, since even though the previous study showed that shape context helped to improve the segmentation accuracy, it is unclear whether that is due to the 3D shape model providing 3D information that is not accessible to 2D U-nets, or to it providing useful context information that will help segmentation.

In comparison with other context approaches such as auto-context, the shape context can eliminate irregularities in the preliminary segmentation results, such as isolated regions outside the targeted bone or holes inside the bone, while the conventional auto-context that will be based only on the output of the first U-net. In another study, we compared several types of context information for deep neural networks and found shape context produced the most accurate results. These findings will be reported in a future publication.

Another contribution of the proposed method is to replace the two sets of U-nets with a single U-net that can take blank shape context channels and introduce an iterative training and testing scheme, which was not reported in the previous work. The iterative scheme not only reduces the file size for deploying the trained net, saving the time of loading and switching network into computer memory, but also makes it possible to run the shape model estimation and shape-context-based segmentation multiple times in an iterative manner. This will hopefully further improve the segmentation accuracy. (However, the benefit of running over 2 passes was not very evident in our experiments.) It is worth noticing the two networks setup proposed in [8], can also be run in an iterative mode by repeating the testing process using the second set of 2D U-nets. Similar performance gain is expected in the 2D cases.

Wang et al. reported overfitting on certain structures when applying their 2.5 U-net with shape context to the heart segmentation, i.e. the segmentation accuracy drops when the shape context is added [8]. The design of trying to use a single 3D U-net to handle cases with and without shape context will force the network to not rely on the shape context too much, avoiding overfitting.

Several strategies were tested to make sure that, after the second-round training, the single 3D U-net can perform well on samples with only the input CT image (with blank shape context channels) and samples with both CT image and shape context channels. These strategies included mixing the training samples with and without shape context, alternating training between two types of training samples, and complete retraining while gradually adding one group into another. However, it was found that simply continuing to train the U-net with samples with shape context works best. As shown in Table 1, the segmentation accuracy of the 1st pass on the retrained 3D U-net is only slightly inferior to the results of the 3D U-net trained on samples without shape context.

One limitation of this study was the lack of diseased cases in the image sample used. The performance must be evaluated where fracture or other abnormality exists. Another limitation was that the down-sampling of the input images due to hardware limitations which introduced additional errors. Finally, the ground-truth segmentation was generated by a single doctor, no inter-observer variation information is available. Future research activities have been planned to address these limitations.

In conclusion, a multi-pass 3D U-net framework with iteratively estimated shape models as context information was proposed. Preliminary results show that the proposed method outperforms both 2D and 3D conventional U-nets in 3D pelvis segmentation.

**Acknowledgements.** This study was supported by the Swedish Heart-lung foundation (grant no. 20160609), Swedish Medtech4Health AIDA research grant, and the Swedish Childhood Cancer Foundation (grant no. MT2016-00166).

# References

1. Seim, H., Kainmüller, D., Heller, M., Lamecker, H., Zachow, S., Hege, H.C.: Automatic segmentation of the pelvic bones from CT data based on a statistical shape model. In: Proceedings 1st Eurographics Conference on Visual Computing for Biomedicine - EG VCBM 2008, pp. 93–100 (2008). https://doi.org/10.2312/VCBM/VCBM08/093-100
2. Kang, Y., Engelke, K., Kalender, W.: A new accurate and precise 3-D segmentation method for skeletal structures in volumetric CT data. IEEE Trans. Med. Imaging **22**(5), 586–598 (2003). https://doi.org/10.1109/TMI.2003.812265
3. Chu, C., Chen, C., Liu, L., Zheng, G.: FACTS: fully automatic CT segmentation of a hip joint. Ann. Biomed. Eng. **43**(5), 1247–1259 (2015). https://doi.org/10.1007/s10439-014-1176-4
4. Chu, C., Bai, J., Wu, X., Zheng, G.: MASCG: multi-atlas segmentation constrained graph method for accurate segmentation of hip CT images. Med. Image Anal. **26**(1), 173–184 (2015). https://doi.org/10.1016/j.media.2015.08.011
5. Long, J., Shelhamer, E., Darrell, T.: Fully convolutional networks for semantic segmentation. In: Proceedings of IEEE Conference on Computer Vision and Pattern Recognition - CVPR 2015, pp. 3431–3440. IEEE (2015). https://doi.org/10.1109/CVPR.2015.7298965
6. Ronneberger, O., Fischer, P., Brox, T.: U-Net: convolutional networks for biomedical image segmentation. In: Navab, N., Hornegger, J., Wells, W.M., Frangi, A.F. (eds.) MICCAI 2015. LNCS, vol. 9351, pp. 234–241. Springer, Cham (2015). https://doi.org/10.1007/978-3-319-24574-4_28
7. Yokota, F., Okada, T., Takao, M., Sugano, N., Tada, Y., Sato, Y.: Automated segmentation of the femur and pelvis from 3D CT data of diseased hip using hierarchical statistical shape model of joint structure. In: Yang, G.-Z., Hawkes, D., Rueckert, D., Noble, A., Taylor, C. (eds.) MICCAI 2009. LNCS, vol. 5762, pp. 811–818. Springer, Heidelberg (2009). https://doi.org/10.1007/978-3-642-04271-3_98

8. Wang, C., Smedby, Ö.: Automatic whole heart segmentation using deep learning and shape context. In: Pop, M., et al. (eds.) STACOM 2017. LNCS, vol. 10663, pp. 242–249. Springer, Cham (2018). https://doi.org/10.1007/978-3-319-75541-0_26
9. Johnson, C., et al.: Accuracy of CT colonography for detection of large adenomas and cancers. N. Engl. J. Med. **359**(12), 1207–1217 (2008). https://doi.org/10.1056/NEJMoa0800996
10. Roth, H.R., et al.: A new 2.5D representation for lymph node detection using random sets of deep convolutional neural network observations. In: Golland, P., Hata, N., Barillot, C., Hornegger, J., Howe, R. (eds.) MICCAI 2014. LNCS, vol. 8673, pp. 520–527. Springer, Cham (2014). https://doi.org/10.1007/978-3-319-10404-1_65
11. Yushkevich, P., et al.: User-guided 3D active contour segmentation of anatomical structures: significantly improved efficiency and reliability. Neuroimage **31**(3), 1116–1128 (2006). https://doi.org/10.1016/j.neuroimage.2006.01.015
12. Leventon, M., Grimson, W., Faugeras, O.: Statistical shape influence in geodesic active contours. In: Proceedings of IEEE Conference on Computer Vision and Pattern Recognition - CVPR 2000, pp. 316–323. IEEE (2000). https://doi.org/10.1109/CVPR.2000.855835
13. Wang, C., Smedby, Ö.: Automatic multi-organ segmentation in non-enhanced CT datasets using hierarchical shape priors. In: Proceedings of 22nd International Conference on Pattern Recognition - ICPR 2014, pp. 3327–3332. IEEE (2014). https://doi.org/10.1109/ICPR.2014.574

# Bone Adaptation as Level Set Motion

Bryce A. Besler[1,2,4(✉)], Leigh Gabel[2,4], Lauren A. Burt[2,4], Nils D. Forkert[3,4], and Steven K. Boyd[2,4]

[1] Biomedical Engineering Graduate Program, University of Calgary, Calgary, Canada
babesler@ucalgary.ca
[2] McCaig Institute for Bone and Joint Health, University of Calgary, Calgary, Canada
[3] Hotchkiss Brain Institute, University of Calgary, Calgary, Canada
[4] Department of Radiology, Cumming School of Medicine, University of Calgary, Calgary, Canada

**Abstract.** Bone microarchitecture is constantly adapting to environmental and mechanical factors. Changes in bone density and structure can lead to an increase in fracture risk. Computational modeling of bone adaptation may provide insight into mitigating aging and preventing disease. In this paper, the adaptation of bone is modeled as a curve evolution problem. Curves can be evolved according to the level set method. The level set method models basic bone physiology by adapting bone according to appositional growth following a trajectory in time with a natural definition of homeostasis. A novel curvature based bone adaptation algorithm is presented for modeling bone atrophy. The algorithm is shown to be weakly equivalent to simulated bone atrophy. These results generalize surface-driven and strain-driven models of bone adaptation using a surface remodeling force. Physiological signals (hormones, mechanical strain, etc.) can be directly integrated into this surface remodeling force. Remodeling can be naturally restricted around foreign bodies (such as modeling adaptation around a surgical screw). Future work aims to identify the surface remodeling force from longitudinal image data.

**Keywords:** Level set method · Bone adaptation · Cancellous bone · Finite difference method

## 1 Introduction

Bone is a dynamic organ changing shape and density in time. Constantly, bone is undergoing a process of remodeling, where cellular processes remove old bone and lay down new bone [1]. Bone adaptation is driven by many factors, including genetics, hormones, and mechanical loading [2]. An imbalance in resorption and formation can lead to a degradation of bone microarchitecture, increasing the risk of fracture. Computational modeling of bone adaptation can provide insight into aging and metabolic bone diseases such as osteoporosis.

© Springer Nature Switzerland AG 2019
T. Vrtovec et al. (Eds.): MSKI 2018, LNCS 11404, pp. 58–72, 2019.
https://doi.org/10.1007/978-3-030-11166-3_6

In this paper, the physiological process of bone adaptation is modeled using level set motion. In Sect. 2, a framework is presented for modeling bone adaptation as a curve evolution problem. Bone physiology and curve evolution are reviewed and used to derive a surface-only model of bone atrophy based on mean curvature and advection. In Sect. 3, numerical techniques for solving the partial differential equation are summarized. In Sect. 4, quadratic surfaces are used to demonstrate that the algorithm produces physiologically plausible changes. Finally, in Sect. 5, curvature based bone adaptation is shown to generalize a classic surface-driven model of bone atrophy using *in vivo* image data.

## 2   Bone Adaptation as Level Set Motion

Cancellous bone is a mixture of marrow tissue and trabeculae tissue. Bone can only remodel at the surface – so-called appositional growth [1]. The interface between marrow tissue and trabeculae tissue defines a surface. Remodeling of bone microarchitecture can be conceptualized as an evolution of this surface.

### 2.1   Bone Microarchitecture as a Curve

First, the trabecular surface is modeled by a planar curve $\mathcal{C}$, which maps the normalized length along the curve to a two-dimensional coordinate:

$$\mathcal{C} : [0, 1] \rightarrow \mathbb{R}^2. \tag{1}$$

The curve requires an explicit parameterization, which is typically realized using splines [3]. The curve can be evolved in time along its normal vector $\boldsymbol{N}$ according to a force $F$:

$$\mathcal{C}_t = F\boldsymbol{N}, \tag{2}$$

where $\mathcal{C}_t$ is the time derivative of the curve. Importantly, the force $F$ can depend on mean curvature, $\kappa$. This definition of a curve is inherently limited to planar curves. Furthermore, parameterized curves cannot change topology without explicit breaking and merging rules.

Alternatively, a curve can be defined as the level set of an embedding function [4]. Let $\phi$ be an N-dimensional image defined on domain $\Omega \in \mathbb{Z}^n$ and map each point $x \in \Omega$ to $\mathbb{R}$. The curve $\mathcal{C}$ is defined as the zero level set of the embedding function $\phi$:

$$\mathcal{C} = \{x | x \in \Omega, \phi(x) = 0\}. \tag{3}$$

The level set may be evolved by some force, $F$, by noting that (3) must hold for all time [5]:

$$\phi\left(\mathcal{C}(t), t\right) = 0. \tag{4}$$

By differentiating (4) with respect to time, the following equation of motion for N-dimensional curves is found:

$$\phi_t + F|\nabla\phi| = 0. \tag{5}$$

Similar to (2), the force $F$ may depend on mean curvature, $\kappa$. Curvature can be computed directly from the embedding image $\phi$ as the divergence of the normal vectors to the curve [6]:

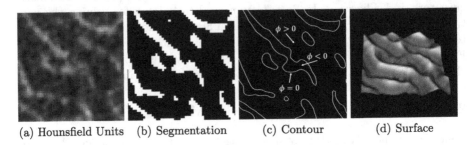

(a) Hounsfield Units    (b) Segmentation    (c) Contour    (d) Surface

**Fig. 1.** Embedding computed tomography data in a level set. Although a two-dimensional image is shown, the embedding is done on three-dimensional data.

$$\kappa = \nabla \cdot \boldsymbol{N}, \tag{6}$$

$$\kappa = \nabla \cdot \left( \frac{\nabla \phi}{|\nabla \phi|} \right). \tag{7}$$

There are many possible choices of $\phi$. Here, $\phi$ is defined as the signed distance between a voxel and the curve:

$$\phi(x) = \pm d\left(x, \mathcal{C}\right). \tag{8}$$

The distance $\pm d\left(x, \mathcal{C}\right)$ is a signed Euclidean distance such that $d < 0$ is inside the curve and $d > 0$ is outside the curve. The image $\phi$ can be computed in linear time from a binarized image of cancellous bone [7]. Figure 1 demonstrates the concept of embedding trabecular bone in a level set.

The level set formulation of curve evolution has many advantages. First, the definition is non-parametric. More precisely, the curve is implicitly parameterized by the domain of the image instead of relying on a parameterization such as splines. Second, the level set method implicitly handles changes in topology. This is important for modeling the resorption of trabecular bone because thin trabecular rods can completely resorb, changing the topology of the bone [8].

## 2.2   Functional Adaptation as Curve Evolution

Functional bone adaptation is defined as the ability of bone to form or resorb according to local mechanical strain [9]. The curve force $F$ of functional bone adaptation is a surface remodeling rate modulated by local physiological signals (e.g. mechanical strain, hormones, etc.) [2]. Micro-computed tomography can resolve individual trabeculae (on the order of 100 μm) in three dimensions (3D) enabling visualization and quantification of bone adaptation [10,11]. The cancellous bone can be binarized using a density threshold on the computed tomography data. Using finite element modeling [12] with an assumed loading condition, strain energy density can be computed at each voxel. Relating strain energy density to surface remodeling rate gives the curve force $F$ in (5) [13]. Although finite element modeling is not performed in the following experiments, it is important to recognize that the level set method is a general framework for modeling strain- and surface-based bone adaptation.

Importantly, these models present bone adaptation as an initial value problem:

$$\begin{cases} \dfrac{\partial \phi(x,t)}{\partial t} = -F|\nabla \phi(x,t)|, \\ \phi(x,0) = \phi_0(x). \end{cases} \tag{9}$$

The initial value problem implies that bone adapts according to a trajectory in time. Knowing the state of the bone at time $t_0$ and knowledge of how bone functionally adapts (by force $F$ at the surface), a unique solution can be found for all $t$. Furthermore, the curve stops updating when the force $F$ goes to zero (that is, $\phi_t = 0$). This implies a state of homeostasis, important for modeling metabolic diseases such as osteoporosis [14]. The surface remodeling rate $F$ is the fundamental measure needed to understand functional bone adaptation [15–17].

## 2.3   Bone Adaptation by Advection and Mean Curvature

Surface-based models of bone adaptation are important for understanding longitudinal changes in trabecular bone. One such model was simulated bone atrophy (SIBA) [8], where one iteration of the remodeling cycle was simulated at a time. The basis of this approach was that bone remodeling occurs in discrete packets termed Basic Multicellular Units (BMUs). In one remodeling cycle, a BMU is recruited, osteoclast cells resorb bone mineral, and osteblast cells replace this bone in a sequential fashion [1]. Given a binary image of bone, SIBA simulates one remodeling cycle using a Gaussian blur, where a finite impulse response Gaussian filter smooths the edges of the binary image data producing a greyscale image. Subsequently applying a threshold, the greyscale data could be re-binarized. The Gaussian filter standard deviation and support were chosen on the basis of osteoclast penetration depth. The threshold was chosen based on osteoblast efficiency, or percentage of bone resorbed by osteoclasts that osteoblasts replaced, and the time between iterations was chosen as the activation frequency of BMUs. SIBA can be viewed as a net advection and curvature-based loss when a threshold less than 50% is chosen and Gaussian smoothing is included. The approach we present reframes SIBA in the level set motion framework. This is a novel method for modeling age-related bone loss, and importantly unifies surface-based and strain-based models of bone adaptation.

As in Sect. 2.1, consider a curve, $\mathcal{C}$, defining the marrow-trabecular interface. To model appositional growth, one seeks to adapt this curve in time by some force $F$ in the direction of the normal to the curve:

$$\mathcal{C}_t = F\mathbf{N}. \tag{10}$$

In 3D, the curve can be seen as the level set of an embedding function $\phi$. An equation of motion for the curve can be found:

$$\phi_t + F|\nabla\phi| = 0. \tag{11}$$

The force is chosen to have an advection and curvature loss:

$$F = a - b\kappa. \tag{12}$$

By selecting $a$ positive, the curve will grow, increasing the trabecular bone volume. Conversely, negative $a$ causes the curve to shrink, decreasing the trabecular bone volume. The curvature term is only well-posed for $b$ positive [6]. $a$ is measured in units of $\mu$m/year and $b$ is measured in units of $\mu$m$^2$/year. Combining (11) and (12), an equation of motion for the trabecular bone surface can be found:

$$\phi_t = b\kappa|\nabla\phi| - a|\nabla\phi|. \tag{13}$$

Finally, the curve evolution problem can be formulated as an initial value problem by taking $\phi_0(x)$ as the signed Euclidean distance transform of binarized computed tomography data:

$$\begin{cases} \dfrac{\partial\phi(x,t)}{\partial t} = b\kappa|\nabla\phi(x,t)| - a|\nabla\phi(x,t)|, \\ \phi(x,0) = \phi_0(x). \end{cases} \tag{14}$$

Most importantly, the parameters $a$ and $b$ must be selected to represent physiologically plausible change. As with SIBA, the majority of the loss should be accounted for by mean curvature [8]. For this reason, $b\kappa$ should be chosen on the same order or larger in magnitude than $a$. Average loss may provide some insight into the absolute scale of the parameters. For idealized cylindrical rods, the mean curvature is known to be the inverse of twice the radius. Using this, an equation for surface remodeling rate $l$ given a cylinder of radius $r$ can be found:

$$l(r) = a - b\kappa = a - \frac{b}{2r}. \tag{15}$$

Equation (15) is plotted in Fig. 2. Graphically, Fig. 2 demonstrates that the surface remodeling rate accelerates with time for rod-like structures. The mean thickness of trabecular bone ranges from 150 $\mu$m to 250 $\mu$m [18]. Using this model and knowledge of thickness, the following parameters were selected: $a = -1\,\mu$m/year, $b = 100\,\mu$m$^2$/year. This gives a loss of $-1.5\,\mu$m/year for a 100 $\mu$m rod. Note that after one year, the radius decreases and the rate increases in accordance with (15) and Fig. 2. This leads to a cascading loss.

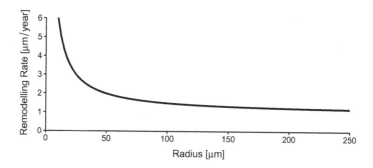

**Fig. 2.** Plot of surface remodeling rate as a function of radius for a rod-like structure ($a = -1\,\mu\text{m/year}$, $b = 10\,\mu\text{m}^2/\text{year}$).

---

**Algorithm 1.** Curvature Based Bone Adaptation
___

**Require:** $\phi_0$, $a$, $b > 0$, $t > 0$
1: $\phi = \phi_0$
2: elapsed $= 0$
3: **while** elapsed $< t$ **do**
4:    $\phi = \text{Reinitialize}(\phi)$
5:    dt $= \min (t$ - elapsed, TimeStep(a,b,$\phi$) )
6:    **for all** $x \in \Omega$ **do**
7:       update $= b$ CurvatureTerm($\phi(x)$) - $a$ AdvectionTerm(a, $\phi(x)$)
8:       $\phi(x) = \phi(x) +$ dt · update
9:    **end for**
10:   elapsed $+=$ dt
11: **end while**
12: **return** $\phi$

---

## 3   Numerical Implementation

The finite difference method is employed to numerically solve (14). Time and space discretization are described in detail below. Since trabecular bone surface is dense in the image domain, narrow band methods are not employed [6]. The algorithm takes an initial distance transform $\phi_0$, the advection and mean curvature weights $a$ and $b$, and a total time to iterate $t$ and returns the final embedded level set. A multithreaded implementation written in C++ and based on The Insight Segmentation and Registration Toolkit[1] is available online[2]. The program is summarized in Algorithm 1. In the following sections, the algorithm is applied to idealized surfaces and *in vivo* image data.

---

[1] www.itk.org.
[2] https://github.com/Bonelab/Bone_Adaptation_as_Level_Set_Motion.

## 3.1   Time Discretization

The forward Euler method can be used for time discretization. However, the spatial discretization of mean curvature and advection require special care [4]:

$$\phi(x, t + \Delta t) = \phi(x, t) + \Delta t \left[ b\kappa |\nabla \phi(x, t)| - a |\nabla \phi(x, t)| \right]. \tag{16}$$

## 3.2   Advection Term

The advection term will be spatially discretized using the upwind scheme [4]. Let $\phi_i \equiv \frac{\partial \phi(x, t)}{\partial x_i}$ denote the derivative of $\phi$ with respect to direction $x_i$. The gradient magnitude can be written as such:

$$|\nabla \phi(x, t)| = \sqrt{\sum_i \phi_i^2}. \tag{17}$$

An upwind finite difference method is used to compute the first order partial derivatives. This is done by calculating the derivative on the edge to which the wave moves. This scheme is known to capture shocks in the evolving wave front. First, forward edge and backwards edge derivative operators are defined:

$$D_i^+ \phi = \frac{\phi_{i+1,j,k} - \phi_{i,j,k}}{\Delta x_i}, \tag{18}$$

$$D_i^- \phi = \frac{\phi_{i,j,k} - \phi_{i-1,j,k}}{\Delta x_i}. \tag{19}$$

The squared partial derivative is estimated by taking into account the direction of wave propagation:

$$\phi_i^2 = \begin{cases} \max \left( D_i^- \phi, 0 \right)^2 + \min \left( D_i^+ \phi, 0 \right)^2, & \text{if } a \geq 0, \\ \min \left( D_i^- \phi, 0 \right)^2 + \max \left( D_i^+ \phi, 0 \right)^2, & \text{if } a < 0. \end{cases} \tag{20}$$

## 3.3   Curvature Term

The curvature term is spatially discretized using central differences [6]. The curvature can be calculated from the level set as the divergence of the normal:

$$\kappa = \nabla \cdot \mathbf{N}, \tag{21}$$

$$\kappa = \nabla \cdot \left( \frac{\nabla \phi}{|\nabla \phi|} \right), \tag{22}$$

$$\kappa = \frac{\Delta \phi}{|\nabla \phi|} - \frac{1}{|\nabla \phi|^3} \sum_i \sum_j \phi_i \phi_j \phi_{ij}, \tag{23}$$

where $\triangle \phi = \nabla \cdot \nabla \phi$ denotes the Laplacian of $\phi$ and $\phi_{i,j} \equiv \frac{\partial^2 \phi(x, t)}{\partial x_i \partial x_j}$ denotes the second derivative of $\phi$ with respect to $x_i$, $x_j$. Using (23) and assuming $\phi$ has continuous derivatives such that $\phi_{ij} = \phi_{ji}$, the mean curvature term can then be reduced to the following:

$$\kappa|\nabla\phi(x,t)| = |\nabla\phi|\left(\frac{\Delta\phi}{|\nabla\phi|} - \frac{1}{|\nabla\phi|^3}\sum_i\sum_j\phi_i\phi_j\phi_{ij}\right), \tag{24}$$

$$\kappa|\nabla\phi(x,t)| = \frac{1}{|\nabla\phi|^2}\left(\sum_i\phi_i^2\sum_{j\neq i}\phi_{jj} - 2\sum_i\sum_{j=i+1}\phi_i\phi_j\phi_{ij}\right). \tag{25}$$

The derivatives in (25) are discretized using central differences since the value depends on cross derivatives in different spatial directions [6]:

$$\phi_i = \frac{\phi_{i+1,j,k} - \phi_{i-1,j,k}}{2\Delta x_i}, \tag{26}$$

$$\phi_{ij} = \begin{cases} \frac{\phi_{i+1,j,k} - 2\phi_{i,j,k} + \phi_{i-1,j,k}}{(\Delta x_i)^2}, \text{if } i = j, \\ \frac{\phi_{i+1,j+1,k} - \phi_{i-1,j+1,k} - \phi_{i+1,j-1,k} + \phi_{i-1,j-1,k}}{4\Delta x_i\Delta x_j}, \text{if } i \neq j. \end{cases} \tag{27}$$

## 3.4   Courant-Friedrichs-Lewy Condition

The level set method provides a strong numerical basis for choosing time steps based on the speed of curve evolution relative to image spacing. The so-called Courant-Friedrichs-Lewy (CFL) condition requires that the numerical domain of dependence includes the analytic domain of dependence [19]. Using an upwind finite difference for the advection term and central differences for the mean curvature term, the following CFL condition must be met for each voxel [6]:

$$\alpha = \Delta t\left(\frac{|a|}{\min\{\Delta x, \Delta y, \Delta z\}} + \frac{2|b|}{\min\{(\Delta x)^2, (\Delta y)^2, (\Delta z)^2\}}\right) < 1. \tag{28}$$

For these experiments, the CFL number was set to a conservative $\alpha = 0.5$ [6].

## 3.5   Reinitialization

Finally, introduction of a mean curvature term with forward Euler time discretization can cause $\phi$ to deviate from a signed distance function. Periodically, reinitialization is needed to return the level set to a signed distance function [6]. The technique used here solves the following reinitialization equation [20]:

$$\phi_t + S(\phi)(|\nabla\phi| - 1) = 0, \tag{29}$$

$$S(\phi) = \frac{\phi}{\sqrt{\phi^2 + |\nabla\phi|^2\epsilon^2}}, \tag{30}$$

where $\epsilon = \min\{\Delta x, \Delta y, \Delta z\}$. Reinitialization updates the embedding function to maintain the property that for a signed distance function, $|\nabla\phi| = 1$. The term $S(\phi)$ is the regularized sign of the embedding function.

# 4    Quadratic Surfaces

To gain insight into the correctness of the resorption algorithm, simple representations of rods and plates will be created using quadratic surfaces. The implicit function of a quadratic surface can be used to instantiate an idealized rod or plate in image data. Below, quadratic surfaces are defined according to physical properties of a rod or plate. The instantiated image data can be created with varying image resolutions, but will not be explored here.

## 4.1    Cylindrical Rod

A rod of constant thickness can be modeled as a cylinder of radius $r$. This rod will have some length $l$, which clips the implicit function:

$$x^2 + y^2 - r^2 = 0. \tag{31}$$

## 4.2    Resorbing Rod

A rod thinning in the center can be modeled as a one sheet hyperbola:

$$b^2 x^2 + b^2 y^2 - a^2 z^2 = 1. \tag{32}$$

The equation is determined by three parameters: the length of the rod, $l$; the radius at the ends of the rod, $R$; and the radius at the center of the rod, $r$:

$$a = \frac{2}{l}\sqrt{\frac{R^2}{r^2} - 1}, \tag{33}$$

$$b = \frac{1}{r}. \tag{34}$$

## 4.3    Resorbing Plate

Finally, a plate can be modeled as a torus. Given below is the equation of a torus:

$$\left(\sqrt{x^2 + y^2} - R\right)^2 + a^2 z^2 = r^2. \tag{35}$$

By varying $R$ with respect to $r$, the size of the hole through the torus can be controlled. If $r > R$, the hole can be closed.

The equation of the torus is determined by three parameters: the diameter of the plate, $l$; the resorption distance, $d$; and the plate thickness, $t$:

$$r = \frac{l - d}{4}, \tag{36}$$

$$R = \frac{l + d}{4}, \tag{37}$$

$$a = \frac{l - d}{2t}. \tag{38}$$

If the resorption distance is negative, the hole in the torus will be closed.

## 4.4    Proof-of-Principle

Three surfaces are generated to visualize the curvature based bone adaptation algorithm. The cases are outlined in Fig. 3. For each case, the implicit functions above are used to generate a representation of the surface in a binary image. The spacing of the images are set to an isotropic resolution of $61\,\mu$m. Fifty years of aging are simulated using the parameters $a = -1\,\mu$m/year and $b = 100\,\mu$m$^2$/year. The surfaces are visualized directly from the embedding function $\phi$ using the Marching Cubes algorithm [21].

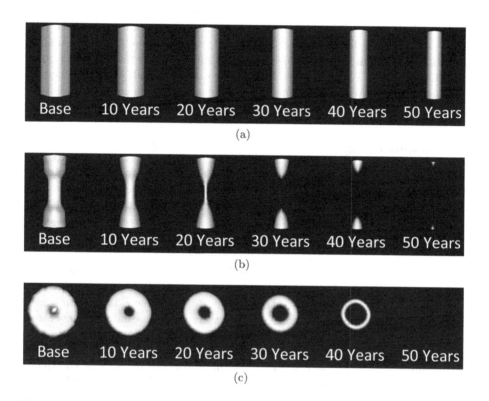

**Fig. 3.** Plot of ideal structures adapting in time. Three cases are demonstrated: (a) Cylindrical rod ($l = 1\,$mm, $r = 200\,\mu$m). (b) Resorbing rod ($l = 1\,$mm, $R = 200\,\mu$m, $r = 100\,$mm). (c) Resorbing plate ($l = 1\,$mm, $d = 100\,$mm, $t = 200\,$mm).

Many important features of the algorithm are demonstrated in Fig. 3. The resorbing rod (Fig. 3(b)) and plate (Fig. 3(c)) are completely removed while the cylindrical rod (Fig. 3(a)) thins. This agrees with the intuition behind (15) and Fig. 2 that higher curvature structures resorb faster. Additionally, the topological change in the resorbing rod is handled implicitly. Handling topolgical changes is a critical feature for any algorithm modeling bone adaptation. Finally, the resorbing plate reduces to a ring. Both the outer and inner portions of the ring resorb. Curvature based bone adaptation demonstrates physiologically plausible changes to idealized rods and plates.

## 5     *In vivo* Experiments

### 5.1     Data Collection

Curvature based bone adaptation is applied to *in vivo* human data as a model of aging. The left, distal tibia of ten subjects were imaged using second generation high-resolution peripheral quantitative computed tomography (HR-pQCT; XtremeCT II, SCANCO Medical AG, Switzerland). Second generation HR-pQCT is capable of directly assessing human trabecular bone [18]. The nominal resolution was 61 μm isotropic. 50% (5) of the subjects were female. Age ranged from 56 to 67 years. Total bone mineral density ranged from 279.6 mg HA/ccm to 317.5 mg HA/ccm. Age- and sex-matched normative total bone mineral density ranged from 48.3% to 53.5% [22].

### 5.2     Pre-processing

Cortical and cancellous masks for each tibia volume were generated using the dual thresholding technique [23]. Masks were visually inspected and manually corrected. Image data was binarized using a threshold of 320 mg HA/ccm.

### 5.3     Simulation

For each subject, 30 years of bone loss was simulated. The simulation parameters were unchanged ($a = -1$ μm/year, $b = 100$ μm$^2$/year). However, a mask of the trabecular bone was included to restrict the remodeling force $F$ to the trabecular region. Outside the trabecular mask, $F$ was set to zero. Image data was generated at every decade, and bone volume fraction in the cancellous compartment was quantified. Additionally, the bone surface area to volume ratio was quantified for the measured data. The surface area to volume ratio is a measure of the shape of the trabecular bone and is a strong determinant of bone loss in SIBA [8]. The surfaces were visualized directly from the embedding function $\phi$ using the Marching Cubes algorithm [21].

### 5.4     Results

The change in morphometry with simulated aging is analyzed. A plot of trabecular bone volume fraction with simulated age is shown in Fig. 4(a). Each subject experiences monotonic bone loss with age. Subjects appear to lose bone at the same absolute rate. This can be explained by having selecting the same parameters ($a$ and $b$) for each subject. Figure 4(b) shows the percent bone loss over 30 years as a function of original bone surface to volume ratio. 99% of the variation in lost bone volume fraction is explained by the original bone surface

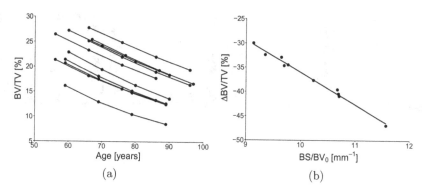

(a)                                    (b)

**Fig. 4.** Change in bone morphometry with simulated age. (a) Trabecular bone volume fraction decreases with simulated age for ten subjects. (b) Original bone surface to bone volume ratio predicts percentage bone loss ($R^2 = 0.99$).

to volume ratio ($p < 0.05$). This is a key finding in the original work on SIBA [8]. Curvature loss for one subject is shown in Figs. 5 and 6. The subject is a 60 year old male with an original bone volume fraction of 22.9% and a bone surface to volume ratio of 10.7 mm$^{-1}$. No loss is seen in the cortical bone where the curve force was set to zero. This is an important feature for modeling complex interactions such as adaptation around a surgical screw. Qualitatively, more bone loss is seen in the center of the bone than the endosteal surface (Fig. 5). This loss visually corresponds with a thin, rod-like initial structure. Plates connected by thin trabecular rods can become disconnected, a feature also present in SIBA. Trabeculae disconnect, holes in plates widen, and loss is seen throughout the structure (Fig. 6). Curvature based bone adaptation appears to model the same mechanism of bone loss as the SIBA algorithm.

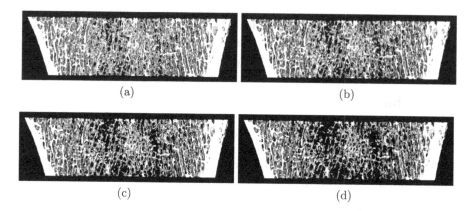

(a)                                    (b)

(c)                                    (d)

**Fig. 5.** Change in microarchitecture under curvature based bone adaptation for one subject at (a) baseline, (b) 10 years, (c) 20 years, and (d) 30 years.

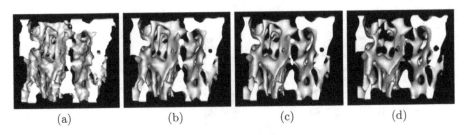

(a)           (b)           (c)           (d)

**Fig. 6.** Microarchitecture loss visualized for a $49 \times 49 \times 49$ ($26.7\,\mu m^3$) volume for one subject at (a) baseline, (b) 10 years, (c) 20 years, and (d) 30 years.

## 6   Discussion

In this paper, bone adaptation is presented as level set motion. Functional adaptation is reviewed in the context of level set motion. A new algorithm for curvature based bone adaptation is presented. This algorithm is shown to generalize simulated bone atrophy using level set motion. The algorithm was applied to idealized structures and *in vivo* image data. Level set methods were previously used to model functional bone adaptation. While one study did not explicitly mention level set motion but derived all components [15], the other only mentioned its use in passing [24]. Level set methods have been well characterized. In general, they can be used to model Hamilton-Jacobi type equations from classical mechanics [4]. Traditionally, bone adaptation is presented as an optimization problem where the bone tries to maintain "mechanical competency" while minimizing mass [2]. However, under level set motion, an interesting future area of research is to reframe bone adaptation using principles of least action.

Finally, level set motion presents a general method for adapting the bone surface according to some force. However, identification of the surface force remains elusive [15–17]. Ideally, the motion force $F$ could be determined uniquely given two longitudinal images. This would allow one to uncover the surface remodeling rate of bone directly from the image data. To the best of our knowledge, very little work towards solving the identification problem has been completed [25, 26].

## 7   Conclusion

Level set motion is a general framework for surface-based and strain-based modeling of bone adaptation. The method matches the basic physiology of bone adaptation: appositional growth. A novel algorithm is presented for modeling bone atrophy using mean curvature and advection.

**Acknowledgements.** B.A. Besler acknowledges support from Alberta Innovates Health Solutions and NSERC CGS-D.

# References

1. Clarke, B.: Normal bone anatomy and physiology. Clin. J. Am. Soc. Nephrol. **3**(Suppl. 3), S131–S139 (2008). https://doi.org/10.2215/CJN.04151206
2. Frost, H.: From Wolff's law to the Utah paradigm: insights about bone physiology and its clinical applications. Anat. Rec. **262**(4), 398–419 (2001). https://doi.org/10.1002/ar.1049
3. Kass, M., Witkin, A., Terzopoulos, D.: Snakes: active contour models. Int. J. Comput. Vis. **1**(4), 321–331 (1988). https://doi.org/10.1007/BF00133570
4. Osher, S., Sethian, J.: Fronts propagating with curvature-dependent speed: algorithms based on Hamilton-Jacobi formulations. J. Comput. Phys. **79**(1), 12–49 (1988). https://doi.org/10.1016/0021-9991(88)90002-2
5. Cremers, D., Rousson, M., Deriche, R.: A review of statistical approaches to level set segmentation: integrating color, texture, motion and shape. Int. J. Comput. Vis. **72**(2), 195–215 (2007). https://doi.org/10.1007/s11263-006-8711-1
6. Osher, S., Fedkiw, R.: Level Set Methods and Dynamic Implicit Surfaces. AMS, vol. 153. Springer, New York (2003). https://doi.org/10.1007/b98879
7. Maurer, C., Qi, R., Raghavan, V.: A linear time algorithm for computing exact Euclidean distance transforms of binary images in arbitrary dimensions. IEEE Trans. Pattern Anal. Mach. Intell. **25**(2), 265–270 (2003). https://doi.org/10.1109/TPAMI.2003.1177156
8. Müller, R.: Long-term prediction of three-dimensional bone architecture in simulations of pre-, peri- and post-menopausal microstructural bone remodeling. Osteoporos. Int. **16**(2), S25–S35 (2005). https://doi.org/10.1007/s00198-004-1701-7
9. Ruff, C., Holt, B., Trinkaus, E.: Who's afraid of the big bad Wolff?: "Wolff's law" and bone functional adaptation. Am. J. Phys. Anthropol. **129**(4), 484–498 (2006). https://doi.org/10.1002/ajpa.20371
10. Rüegsegger, P., Koller, B., Müller, R.: A microtomographic system for the nondestructive evaluation of bone architecture. Calcif. Tissue Int. **58**(1), 24–29 (1996). https://doi.org/10.1007/BF02509542
11. Schulte, F., Lambers, F., Kuhn, G., Müller, R.: In vivo micro-computed tomography allows direct three-dimensional quantification of both bone formation and bone resorption parameters using time-lapsed imaging. Bone **48**(3), 433–442 (2011). https://doi.org/10.1016/j.bone.2010.10.007
12. van Rietbergen, B., Weinans, H., Huiskes, R., Odgaard, A.: A new method to determine trabecular bone elastic properties and loading using micromechanical finite-element models. J. Biomech. **28**(1), 69–81 (1995). https://doi.org/10.1016/0021-9290(95)80008-5
13. Schulte, F., et al.: Strain-adaptive in silico modeling of bone adaptation-a computer simulation validated by in vivo micro-computed tomography data. Bone **52**(1), 485–492 (2013). https://doi.org/10.1016/j.bone.2012.09.008
14. Huiskes, R., Ruimerman, R., Van Lenthe, G., Janssen, J.: Effects of mechanical forces on maintenance and adaptation of form in trabecular bone. Nature **405**(6787), 704–706 (2000). https://doi.org/10.1038/35015116
15. Schulte, F., et al.: Local mechanical stimuli regulate bone formation and resorption in mice at the tissue level. PLoS ONE **8**(4), e62172 (2013). https://doi.org/10.1371/journal.pone.0062172
16. Christen, P., et al.: Bone remodelling in humans is load-driven but not lazy. Nat. Commun. **5**, 4855 (2014). https://doi.org/10.1038/ncomms5855

17. Christen, P., Müller, R.: In vivo visualisation and quantification of bone resorption and bone formation from time-lapse imaging. Curr. Osteoporos. Rep. **15**(4), 311–317 (2017). https://doi.org/10.1007/s11914-017-0372-1

18. Manske, S., Zhu, Y., Sandino, C., Boyd, S.: Human trabecular bone microarchitecture can be assessed independently of density with second generation HR-pQCT. Bone **79**, 213–221 (2015). https://doi.org/10.1016/j.bone.2015.06.006

19. Courant, R., Friedrichs, K., Lewy, H.: Über die partiellen Differenzengleichungen der mathematischen Physik. Math. Ann. **100**(1), 32–74 (1928). https://doi.org/10.1007/BF01448839

20. Peng, D., Merriman, B., Osher, S., Zhao, H., Kang, M.: A PDe-based fast local level set method. J. Comput. Phys. **155**(2), 410–438 (1999). https://doi.org/10.1006/jcph.1999.6345

21. Lorensen, W., Cline, H.: Marching cubes: a high resolution 3D surface construction algorithm. In: Proceedings of 14th Annual Conference on Computer Graphics and Interactive Techniques - SIGGRAPH 1987, pp. 163–169. ACM (1987). https://doi.org/10.1145/37401.37422

22. Burt, L., Liang, Z., Sajobi, T., Hanley, D., Boyd, S.: Sex- and site-specific normative data curves for HR-pQCT. J. Bone Miner. Res. **31**(11), 2041–2047 (2016). https://doi.org/10.1002/jbmr.2873

23. Buie, H., Campbell, G., Klinck, R., MacNeil, J., Boyd, S.: Automatic segmentation of cortical and trabecular compartments based on a dual threshold technique for in vivo micro-CT bone analysis. Bone **41**(4), 505–515 (2007). https://doi.org/10.1016/j.bone.2007.07.007

24. Kameo, Y., Adachi, T.: Modeling trabecular bone adaptation to local bending load regulated by mechanosensing osteocytes. Acta Mech. **225**(10), 2833–2840 (2014). https://doi.org/10.1007/s00707-014-1202-5

25. Yang, I., Tomlin, C.: Identification of surface tension in mean curvature flow. In: Proceedings of 2013 American Control Conference, pp. 3284–3289. IEEE (2013). https://doi.org/10.1109/ACC.2013.6580338

26. Yang, I., Tomlin, C.: Regularization-based identification for level set equations. In: Proceedings of 52nd Annual Conference on Decision and Control - CDC 2013, pp. 1058–1064. IEEE (2013). https://doi.org/10.1109/CDC.2013.6760022

# Landmark Localisation in Radiographs Using Weighted Heatmap Displacement Voting

Adrian K. Davison[1]([✉]), Claudia Lindner[1], Daniel C. Perry[2,3], Weisang Luo[3], Medical Student Annotation Collaborative[2,3], and Timothy F. Cootes[1]

[1] Centre for Imaging Sciences, The University of Manchester, Manchester, UK
`adrian.davison@manchester.ac.uk`
[2] University of Liverpool, Liverpool, UK
[3] Alder Hey Children's Hospital, Liverpool, UK

**Abstract.** We propose a new method for fully automatic landmark localisation using Convolutional Neural Networks (CNNs). Training a CNN to estimate a Gaussian response ("heatmap") around each target point is known to be effective for this task. We show that better results can be obtained by training a CNN to predict the offset to the target point at every location, then using these predictions to vote for the point position. We show the advantages of the approach, including those of using a novel loss function and weighting scheme. We evaluate on a dataset of radiographs of child hips, including both normal and severely diseased cases. We show the effect of varying the training set size. Our results show significant improvements in accuracy and robustness for the proposed method compared to a standard heatmap prediction approach and comparable results with a traditional Random Forest method.

**Keywords:** Perthes disease · X-rays · Paediatrics
Convolutional neural network (CNN)
Fully convolutional network (FCN) · Deep learning · Voting

## 1 Introduction

Locating landmarks on medical images is an important first step in many analysis tasks, particularly those requiring geometric measurements of the shape of structures. Many methods have been proposed for this task, with some of the most effective using random forest regression-voting (RFRV) [1,2] and, more recently, deep learning approaches [3–6].

Deep learning has been a popular method to extract information for classification, recognition and regression tasks. In various fields, convolutional neural networks (CNNs) have become the state-of-the-art, out-performing many traditional machine learning methods. For landmark localisation, including detecting anatomical landmarks in medical images [7,8] and human pose estimation [4,9],

© Springer Nature Switzerland AG 2019
T. Vrtovec et al. (Eds.): MSKI 2018, LNCS 11404, pp. 73–85, 2019.
https://doi.org/10.1007/978-3-030-11166-3_7

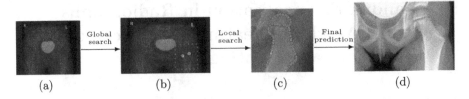

(a)                    (b)                    (c)                    (d)

**Fig. 1.** Overview of our landmark localisation method in child hip radiographs: (a) A full pelvic radiograph. (b) The global searcher network locates two reference points to estimate the pose of the proximal femur. (c) A patch containing the approximately located femur is fed into the local search network to vote for the position of each landmark. (d) The fully automatically predicted landmark positions.

an effective technique has been to apply a CNN to estimate a new image with a Gaussian blob around each predicted landmark position (a so-called "heatmap"). This has been shown to yield better results than directly regressing the landmark locations which tend to have a highly non-linear relationship to features [10].

We propose a novel voting-based scheme to identify landmark locations. We train a fully convolutional NN to estimate the displacement of every pixel from each target landmark, together with an associated weight. These displacements can then be used to vote for the landmark location, integrating information from the local area. We propose a novel loss function to train the CNN for this task, which focuses attention on the target regions. The combination of regressing the pixel offsets and heatmap weights adds further novelty to the approach.

We evaluate the proposed weighted heatmap displacement voting (WHDV) approach on the challenging problem of locating the outline of normal and badly diseased proximal femurs in radiographs of children, showing that WHDV significantly improves both accuracy and robustness compared to a standard heatmap prediction approach. We also show how the performance varies as the number of training examples increases. The overall pipeline can be seen in Fig. 1.

This paper makes three contributions: (i) We describe a novel method of landmark location which improves upon the widely used "heatmap" approach; (ii) we describe extensive experiments characterising the performance of the system as the size of the training set increases. This includes a detailed comparison with random forest regression-voting constrained local models (RFRV-CLMs) demonstrating that unless large numbers of examples are available the latter are to be preferred to CNN approaches; (iii) we demonstrate an automatic system for locating the outline of both normal and diseased femurs, showing that shape model-based systems can deal with considerable abnormalities in this case.

## 2    Related Work

Pfister et al. [4] used a CNN to regress heatmaps for each point, and dense optical flow to warp landmark positions onto videos for human pose estimation. The paper is one of the earliest to regress heatmaps through a deep network and to combine the results with an implicit spatial model.

To detect multiple landmarks on two-dimensional (2D) radiographs and three-dimensional (3D) magnetic resonance imaging (MRI) images of hands, Payer et al. [7] proposed a novel CNN (named SpatialConfiguration-Net) that was trained end-to-end to detect 37 landmarks in the radiographs and 28 in the MRI images. The new architecture could learn local features and imposed constraints on the spatial configuration of landmarks.

Bulat and Tzimiropoulos [9] proposed a CNN cascaded architecture that consisted of two components: a part detection network for detecting human body parts and a deep regression subnetwork that was able to regress the landmark locations using heatmaps, regardless of whether they were occluded or not.

Using the challenging COCO dataset for detecting keypoints, Papandreou et al. [11] used an RCNN detector to find people and estimate keypoints on each using heatmaps and offsets using a fully convolutional ResNet [12]. Both outputs were combined with a novel aggregation function to obtain localised keypoint predictions.

Belagiannis and Zisserman [6] estimated 2D human poses using a CNN with a recurrent module that combined intermediate feature representations to learn the image context and improve the final heatmap predictions in challenging datasets, including those classed as "in-the-wild".

Rather than using heatmaps, the relative position of landmarks can be predicted directly. The majority of such work has focused on medical images. Chen et al. [3] estimated displacements from randomly chosen patches to unknown landmark positions. These patches then voted on the final landmark position. The overall shape was regularised with a statistical shape model.

Aubert et al. [5] used a simple CNN to predict the 3D landmark of vertebral centres. The training used frontal and lateral hip patches to estimate the 2D displacement in the $x$ plane for the frontal and lateral view and for the overall displacement in the $y$ plane. The 3D landmark was determined using epipolar geometry.

Sofka et al. [13] used a fully convolutional network (FCN) to regress point locations. They created a center of mass layer that computed the mean position of the network prediction output. This had an advantage over direct heatmap regression as it could predict subpixel values and the objective function could penalise measurement length differences from the ground truth for their task. This differs from our approach as we calculate the landmark positions outside of the network (with a voting scheme) and we do not need a separate layer to specifically do this task.

Using limited medical image training data, Zhang et al. [8] extracted millions of images patches to be fed into a two-stage convolutional network that first output the predicted displacement vectors, and then directly predicted 1200 landmarks in 3D MRI brain scans and 7 landmarks from 3D tomography images of prostates.

Less common is a combination of heatmaps and displacements. Zhang et al. [14] proposed the use of displacement maps to explicitly model the spatial context information of cone-beam computed tomography scans. They used the estimated displacement maps from the previous step as a guide to introduce a joint learning framework for bone segmentation and landmark localisation. The heatmaps were regressed in the second stage as the ground truth landmark areas.

## 3    Fully Convolutional Network with Global and Local Searchers

Our fully automated method has two stages: (i) a global search over the whole image for two reference points on the target object, which then define its position, orientation and scale; (ii) a local search in a region defined by these reference points to find $n$ landmark points on the object. Both global and local search use the same approach to identify point positions.

We use two separate search stages as a full pelvic X-ray contains many similar features, especially when it comes to the opposite hip. The global search aims to find the position of the left-anatomical femur to then improve the local search performance. Using two reference points to crop the region of interest, in this case the femur, is an established technique to reduce the search area of a potentially cluttered radiograph [1]. To summarise the differences between the global and local searcher: the global searcher scans the whole pelvic X-ray for two key reference points and crops the detected femur; the local searcher uses the cropped image to locate 58 landmark points in a local region of the overall radiograph.

In each case we use a CNN to take the target image (for global search) or sampled region (for local search) and compute a set of output planes for each point. In the original "heatmap" approach one would compute a single image plane for each point. In our modified version we predict three planes per point, an $x$ displacement, a $y$ displacement and a weight plane. We use these to vote for the position of each point and take the maximum response in the accumulated vote image as the final point location.

### 3.1    Convolutional Network with Weighted Heatmap Loss

We use a modified version of the widely used U-Net architecture [15]. U-Net acts as a convolutional auto-encoder with added skip connections from encoder layers to decoder layers that are on the same level. Our modifications are in line with those in [7], where max pooling is replaced with average pooling and up-convolution layers are replaced with upsampling. Our method is similar to [11] in that it uses heatmaps and displacement vectors, however our approach differs by using a vote from every pixel to determine the landmark rather than using probability of being within a disk surrounding a keypoint. Further, we do not require pre-training and use a computationally simpler network architecture, U-net, over the ResNet-101 [12] pretrained on Imagenet.

**Training.** For each input image (with known landmark positions, $(x_p, y_p)$, $p = 1, \ldots, n$), we constructed three ground truth planes $P_x^p$, $P_y^p$, $P_w^p$ as follows:

$$
\begin{aligned}
P_x^p(i,j) &= t(i - x_p), \\
P_y^p(i,j) &= t(j - y_p), \\
P_w^p(i,j) &= \exp(-|(i,j) - (x_p, y_p)|^2 / 2\sigma^2).
\end{aligned}
\tag{1}
$$

The function $t(x)$ truncates the input to a fixed range:

$$
t(x) = \begin{cases}
-k & \text{if } x < -k, \\
k & \text{if } x > k, \\
x & \text{otherwise,}
\end{cases}
\tag{2}
$$

where $k$ is the displacement value chosen through empirical experiments. Note that $P_w^p$ is the traditional "heatmap", a Gaussian blob centred on the landmark. $P_x$ and $P_y$ are displacement planes and $\sigma$ is the standard deviation of the Gaussian function.

We trained the CNN to predict these $3n$ planes for each training image, using a loss function which encourages accurate displacement predictions near the points:

$$
LossPerPixel(\hat{P}_w^p, \hat{P}_x^p, \hat{P}_y^p) = P_w^p((P_x^p - \hat{P}_x^p)^2 + (P_y^p - \hat{P}_y^p)^2)) + (P_w^p - \hat{P}_w^p)^2, \tag{3}
$$

where $\hat{P}_w^p, \hat{P}_x^p, \hat{P}_y^p$ are the outputs of the network. Note that scaling the first term by $P_w^p$ down-weights the position prediction away from the points, where it is not needed.

**Point Localisation.** To locate points on a new image, we feed the image to the CNN to generate the predicted planes. For each point $p$ we then create a vote image, $V_p$, by scanning through all pixels $(i,j)$, voting at $(i + \hat{P}_x^p(i,j), j + \hat{P}_y^p(i,j))$. The vote image is then multiplied (pixel-wise) by the weight image $\hat{P}_w^p(i,j)$. We smooth the vote image with a Gaussian with a SD $= 4$, which was chosen through experiments by changing the SD from 1...6 and choosing the best performing value. The maximum peak of the vote image is used to estimate the point positions.

## 4    Experiments

We performed a series of experiments to accurately locate landmarks along the proximal femur in radiographs of children's hips. To evaluate the performance of the proposed WHDV approach, we compare with two FCN heatmap-based approaches and a traditional machine learning method: RFRV [1,2].

### 4.1 Dataset

The dataset consists of 1,696 radiographs of hips from children aged between 2 and 11 years, with some affected by Perthes disease, where the blood supply to the growth plate of the bone at the end of the femur becomes inadequate [16]. This dataset is challenging as the hip is still growing during childhood, meaning the femur has growth areas such as the femoral head and greater trochanter, and because there is significant shape and appearance change due to disease (Fig. 2(b)).

We conducted 3-fold cross-validation experiments for a range of training set sizes, splitting the data into random subsets of 100, 200, 500 and 1000. The test data consists of 500 randomly chosen images (the same set used for all experiments). The test data does not overlap with the training data for any of the subsets. All images have been manually annotated with 58 points by two different people chosen randomly from a pool of ten trained annotators. The ground truth is then created by averaging the point positions between the two annotators.

For the deep learning based approaches, the data was augmented with random rotations (between 5° clockwise and 35° anti-clockwise) once for each image to allow for rotation variants (note that RFRV also includes random rotations as part of the training). The reason for the imbalance in rotation values is that rotating the hip too far clockwise would create an unrealistic pose for a pelvic X-ray.

### 4.2 Network Parameters

Our FCN takes input images of size $256 \times 192$ (global search) or $224 \times 224$ (local search) and generates $3n$ output planes of the same size as described above. During training, 15% of the training set is used for validation. To ensure the validation set did not use a portion of the training set, we added 15% additional images to the training set. We performed 3-fold cross-validation experiments per method, where the reported results will show the average over all 3 folds.

We chose the Adam [17] optimiser through empirical experiments where all of the available optimisers in Keras (including stochastic gradient descent, Nadam and RMSProp) were tested with the network and the best performing chosen. We used the default parameters suggested in [17], where the learning rate was set to 0.001, the exponential decay rate for the first moment estimates ($\beta_1$) was set to 0.9 and the exponential decay rate for the second-moment estimates ($\beta_2$) was set to 0.999. To prevent division by zero, $\epsilon$ was set to $10^{-7}$. The batch size was set to 10 and training was completed using an NVIDIA Titan Xp GPU. We use Keras [18] with a Tensorflow [19] backend.

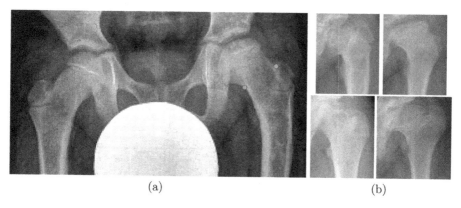

(a)                                                    (b)

**Fig. 2.** (a) Two reference points were chosen to train the global searcher to locate the left proximal femur. Note that the input image is a full pelvic image, adding to the detection difficulty. (b) Sample images from the dataset showing the challenging nature of the diseased proximal femurs.

### 4.3    Global Search

We focused on detecting the left proximal femur in full pelvic images. Each image was scaled to $192 \times 256$ along with 2 ground truth reference points (Fig. 2(a)). Each image was fed into the weighted heatmap loss network with the 3 ground truth elements $(P_x^p, P_y^p, P_w^p)$. The network was trained to regress heatmaps and displacements for the two reference points, and landmark voting was applied to estimate their position. The latter was then used to sample the region of interest for the point localisation stage.

The two reference points were used to define the location, scale and orientation of a region of interest around the proximal femur which was sampled into a $224 \times 224$ patch. Such patches were used to train the second local search CNN to estimate the position of all 58 points.

### 4.4    Landmark Localisation Results

We investigated three CNN based methods: (i) The "Heatmap Only" (HO) approach where the network learns a heatmap centred on each landmark, trained using a mean squared error (MSE) loss; (ii) The "Heatmap with Displacement Voting" (HDV) method where we learned displacement and weight planes using an MSE loss; and (iii) the full WHDV approach with novel weighted loss function. The HO approach is based on the standard heatmap generation [10]. We note that other methods based around this, for example stacked hourglass networks [20], use heatmaps with a more sophisticated network structure, however we use the basic form of heatmap regression in this paper.

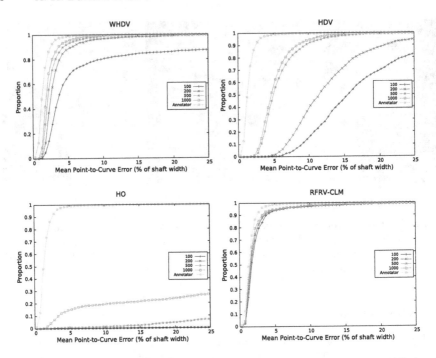

**Fig. 3.** The cumulative distribution functions of mean point-to-curve error for each method as a function of training set size.

We report both mean point-to-curve and mean point-to-point errors measured as a percentage of the femoral shaft width defined by the distance between the bottom two landmark points (Fig. 1(d)). For comparison, we include results using the current state-of-the-art approach, a RFRV-CLM [1,2] which uses random forests with Haar features to vote on the most likely landmark position, constrained using a shape model. We evaluated the accuracy with which the data was annotated by comparing results of 2 independent annotators on 1,696 images. We compute the average difference of each set of annotated points to the mean of the annotations for each image. This gives an indication of the maximum accuracy that may be achieved given the noise on the annotations (see curves marked "Annotator" on the graphs).

Firstly, we show the cumulative distribution function (CDF) graphs for all methods with the mean point-to-curve and point-to-point error for each training size in Figs. 3 and 4 respectively. For WHDV and HDV, the error is reduced as the training size grows, however WHDV performs better than the other 'heatmap'approaches even with a small training set, suggesting the novel loss function helps to stabilise the error, unlike in the similar HDV method. The increase in training data for the proposed method has a particular impact in the point-to-point error going from a median error of 12.5% in the 100 train set, to 6.71% in the 1000 train set.

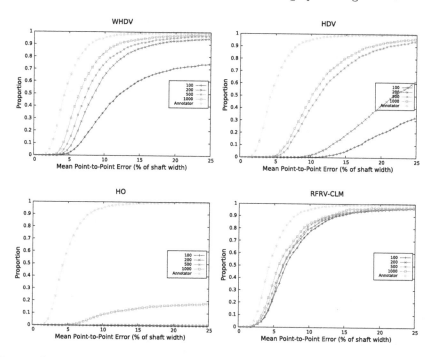

**Fig. 4.** The cumulative distribution functions of mean point-to-point error for each method as a function of training set size.

In contrast, the RFRV-CLM method performs well for all training set sizes, however, unlike the other methods only shows small increases in performance, suggesting that adding more data would not effect the performance as much as it would in the proposed method. For example, the median error in the 100 train set and the 1000 train set was 6.92% and 5.85% respectively for the RFRV-CLM.

A comparison of each method, split into the four training set sizes for both point-to-curve and point-to-point error (Figs. 5 and 6, respectively). These results show that the HO approach performs poorly, regardless of the amount of training data, suggesting that the initial global search fails to locate the hip, which leads to poor performance of the local searcher.

The proposed method is outperformed by RFRV-CLM when trained on only 100 images. However the performance gap closes rapidly as more images are used for training. When trained with 500 examples WHDV outperforms RFRV-CLM significantly in the 99%ile with WHDV achieving a mean point-to-curve error of 10.6% and RFRV-CLM achieving 17.2%. With 1000 images WHDV and RFRV-CLM achieve a mean point-to-curve error of 9.02% and 17.1% respectively. Thus with larger training sets WHDV is more robust (making fewer large errors) than the RFRV-CLM.

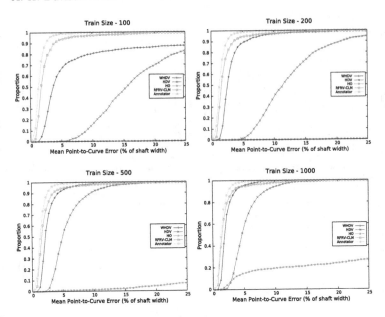

**Fig. 5.** The cumulative distribution function comparing the performance of each method by the training set size. The mean point-to-curve error is reported.

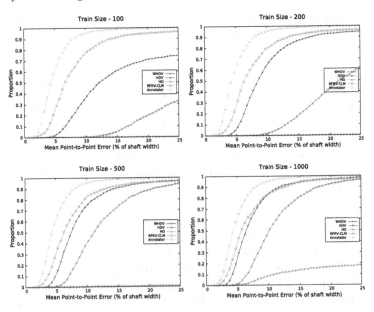

**Fig. 6.** The cumulative distribution function comparing the performance of each method by the training set size. The mean point-to-point error is reported.

# 5   Conclusion

We have described a novel voting-based heatmap method for training CNNs to identify the position of landmark points. Our results show that the proposed method leads to more accurate and robust results than the commonly used "standard heatmap" [10] approach on a challenging data set. One limitation of the voting approach is that it cannot easily be differentiated. This would prohibit full end-to-end training of any system using this approach as its first stage. We showed extensive experiments in characterising the performance of the system as training set sizes increase, which included a comparison with the RFRV-CLM. The experiments showed that unless large numbers of training data can be used, the latter system is to be preferred over CNN approaches. Finally, we demonstrated an automatic system to locate the outline of both normal and diseased femurs, showing the effectiveness of shape-model systems when presented with considerable abnormalities.

RFRV-CLM is a mature technology and is known to work well even on relatively small datasets. It also has the advantage of constraining the points with an explicit (linear) shape model. However, it can be seen that as training data increases, RFRV-CLM has only modest increases in performance. The proposed WHDV method performs poorly when trained on few examples, but outperforms RFRV-CLM in the upper percentiles of the 500 and 1000 train set sizes. Splitting the data into disease and healthy cases would also be useful, but would require clinical expertise to classify the ground truth. Further work will include acquisition of larger datasets with a good representation of healthy and diseased cases, and more analysis on individual age groups and their affect on performance.

The CNN, being trained on all points at once, should learn an implicit model, but some of the errors it makes suggest that this model may not be generalising as well as the traditional RF approach constrained with a shape model – this is something we continue to explore. We will also evaluate whether fitting a shape model to the voting images produces better results, though examination of the votes in the response images suggests that this might not be the case.

Both WHDV and RFRV-CLM perform well in automatically locating landmark points and the outline of the proximal femurs of children, both in cases with and without disease. When starting a new project of this nature, one will only have a few annotated images at first - the RFRV-CLM is much more suitable for helping annotators when building up the training set. This is the first step in the development of a system to quantify shape changes due to disease and to assist clinicians in the decision making on the best course of treatment.

**Acknowledgements.** A. K. Davison was funded by Arthritis Research UK as part of the ORCHiD project. C. Lindner was funded by the Engineering and Physical Sciences Research Council, UK (EP/M012611/1) and by the Medical Research Council, UK (MR/S00405X/1). Manual landmark annotations were provided by the Medical Student Annotation Collaborative (Grace Airey, Evan Araia, Aishwarya Avula, Emily Gargan, Mihika Joshi, Muhammad Khan, Kantida Koysombat, Jason Lee, Sophie Munday and Allen Roby).

# References

1. Lindner, C., Thiagarajah, S., Wilkinson, J., The arcOGEN Consortium, Wallis, G., Cootes, T.: Fully automatic segmentation of the proximal femur using random forest regression voting. IEEE Trans. Med. Imag. **32**(8), 1462–1472 (2013). https://doi.org/10.1109/TMI.2013.2258030

2. Lindner, C., Bromiley, P., Ionita, M., Cootes, T.: Robust and accurate shape model matching using random forest regression-voting. IEEE Trans. Pattern Anal. Mach. Intell. **37**(9), 1862–1874 (2015). https://doi.org/10.1109/TPAMI.2014.2382106

3. Chen, C., Xie, W., Franke, J., Grutzner, P., Nolte, L., Zheng, G.: Automatic X-ray landmark detection and shape segmentation via data-driven joint estimation of image displacements. Med. Image Anal. **18**(3), 487–499 (2014). https://doi.org/10.1016/j.media.2014.01.002

4. Pfister, T., Charles, J., Zisserman, A.: Flowing ConvNets for human pose estimation in videos. In: International Conference on Computer Vision, ICCV 2015, pp. 1913–1921. IEEE (2015). https://doi.org/10.1109/ICCV.2015.222

5. Aubert, B., Vidal, P.A., Parent, S., Cresson, T., Vazquez, C., De Guise, J.: Convolutional neural network and in-painting techniques for the automatic assessment of scoliotic spine surgery from biplanar radiographs. In: Descoteaux, M., Maier-Hein, L., Franz, A., Jannin, P., Collins, D.L., Duchesne, S. (eds.) MICCAI 2017. LNCS, vol. 10434, pp. 691–699. Springer, Cham (2017). https://doi.org/10.1007/978-3-319-66185-8_78

6. Belagiannis, V., Zisserman, A.: Recurrent human pose estimation. In: Proceedings of 12th International Conference on Automatic Face & Gesture Recognition, FG 2017, pp. 468–475. IEEE (2017). https://doi.org/10.1109/FG.2017.64

7. Payer, C., Štern, D., Bischof, H., Urschler, M.: Regressing heatmaps for multiple landmark localization using CNNs. In: Ourselin, S., Joskowicz, L., Sabuncu, M.R., Unal, G., Wells, W. (eds.) MICCAI 2016. LNCS, vol. 9901, pp. 230–238. Springer, Cham (2016). https://doi.org/10.1007/978-3-319-46723-8_27

8. Zhang, J., Liu, M., Shen, D.: Detecting anatomical landmarks from limited medical imaging data using two-stage task-oriented deep neural networks. IEEE Trans. Image Process. **26**(10), 4753–4764 (2017). https://doi.org/10.1109/TIP.2017.2721106

9. Bulat, A., Tzimiropoulos, G.: Human pose estimation via convolutional part heatmap regression. In: Leibe, B., Matas, J., Sebe, N., Welling, M. (eds.) ECCV 2016. LNCS, vol. 9911, pp. 717–732. Springer, Cham (2016). https://doi.org/10.1007/978-3-319-46478-7_44

10. Tompson, J., Jain, A., LeCun, Y., Bregler, C.: Joint training of a convolutional network and a graphical model for human pose estimation. In: Ghahramani, Z., et al. (eds.) Advances in Neural Information Processing Systems, NIPS Proceedings, vol. 27, pp. 1799–1807 (2014)

11. Papandreou, G., et al.: Towards accurate multi-person pose estimation in the wild. In: Proceedings of IEEE Conference on Computer Vision and Pattern Recognition, CVPR 2017, pp. 3711–3719. IEEE (2017). https://doi.org/10.1109/CVPR.2017.395

12. He, K., Zhang, X., Ren, S., Sun, J.: Deep residual learning for image recognition. In: Proceedings of IEEE Conference on Computer Vision and Pattern Recognition, CVPR 2016, pp. 770–778. IEEE (2016). https://doi.org/10.1109/CVPR.2016.90

13. Sofka, M., Milletari, F., Jia, J., Rothberg, A.: Fully convolutional regression network for accurate detection of measurement points. In: Cardoso, M.J., et al. (eds.) DLMIA/ML-CDS 2017. LNCS, vol. 10553, pp. 258–266. Springer, Cham (2017). https://doi.org/10.1007/978-3-319-67558-9_30

14. Zhang, J., et al.: Joint craniomaxillofacial bone segmentation and landmark digitization by context-guided fully convolutional networks. In: Descoteaux, M., Maier-Hein, L., Franz, A., Jannin, P., Collins, D.L., Duchesne, S. (eds.) MICCAI 2017. LNCS, vol. 10434, pp. 720–728. Springer, Cham (2017). https://doi.org/10.1007/978-3-319-66185-8_81

15. Ronneberger, O., Fischer, P., Brox, T.: U-Net: convolutional networks for biomedical image segmentation. In: Navab, N., Hornegger, J., Wells, W.M., Frangi, A.F. (eds.) MICCAI 2015. LNCS, vol. 9351, pp. 234–241. Springer, Cham (2015). https://doi.org/10.1007/978-3-319-24574-4_28

16. Perry, D., Hall, A.: The epidemiology and etiology of Perthes disease. Orthop. Clin. North Am. **42**(3), 279–283 (2011). https://doi.org/10.1016/j.ocl.2011.03.002

17. Kingma, D., Ba, J.: Adam: a method for stochastic optimization. arXiv:1412.6980 (2014)

18. Keras: deep learning for humans (2015). https://github.com/keras-team/keras

19. TensorFlow: large-scale machine learning on heterogeneous systems (2015). https://www.tensorflow.org

20. Newell, A., Yang, K., Deng, J.: Stacked hourglass networks for human pose estimation. In: Leibe, B., Matas, J., Sebe, N., Welling, M. (eds.) ECCV 2016. LNCS, vol. 9912, pp. 483–499. Springer, Cham (2016). https://doi.org/10.1007/978-3-319-46484-8_29

# Perthes Disease Classification
# Using Shape and Appearance Modelling

Adrian K. Davison[1(✉)], Timothy F. Cootes[1], Daniel C. Perry[2,3], Weisang Luo[3], Medical Student Annotation Collaborative[2,3], and Claudia Lindner[1]

[1] Centre for Imaging Sciences, The University of Manchester, Manchester, UK
adrian.davison@manchester.ac.uk
[2] University of Liverpool, Liverpool, UK
[3] Alder Hey Children's Hospital, Liverpool, UK

**Abstract.** We propose to use statistical shape and appearance modelling to classify the proximal femur in hip radiographs of children into Legg-Calvé-Perthes disease and healthy. Legg-Calvé-Perthes disease affects the femoral head with avascular necrosis, which causes large shape deformities during the growth-stage of the child. Further, the dead or dying bone of the femoral head is prominent visually in radiographic images, leading to a distinction between healthy bone and bone where necrosis is present. Currently, there is little to no research into analysing the shape and appearance of hips affected by Perthes disease from radiographic images. Our research demonstrates how the radiographic shape, texture and overall appearance of a proximal femur affected by Perthes disease differs and how this can be used for identifying cases with the disease. Moreover, we present a radiograph-based fully automatic Perthes classification system that achieves state-of-the-art results with an area under the receiver operator characteristic (ROC) curve of 98%.

**Keywords:** Computer-aided diagnosis · Perthes disease
Random forests · Radiographs · Paediatrics · Shape modelling
Appearance modelling

## 1 Introduction

Legg-Calvé-Perthes disease (Perthes) is an idiopathic disease in children between the ages of 2–14 years, with boys being affected 5 times more than girls [1]. The age-of-onset follows a lognormal distribution i.e. the disease has the tendency to affect younger rather than older children [2,3]. Perthes disease is usually analysed through radiographic images in the anterior-posterior (AP) or frog lateral views of the hip. It is not yet known what exactly causes Perthes disease, however, environmental, congenital and socio-economic issues have been associated with Perthes [4]. There is also currently no defined best practice on how to treat the disease, and the decision is usually determined by the treating surgeon. One way of helping to identify and treat Perthes in clinical practice is to use classification methods. Three main categories exist: classification of the stage of disease

© Springer Nature Switzerland AG 2019
T. Vrtovec et al. (Eds.): MSKI 2018, LNCS 11404, pp. 86–98, 2019.
https://doi.org/10.1007/978-3-030-11166-3_8

progression [5,6], classification of prognostic outcomes [7–9] and classification of the patient's long term outcome [10].

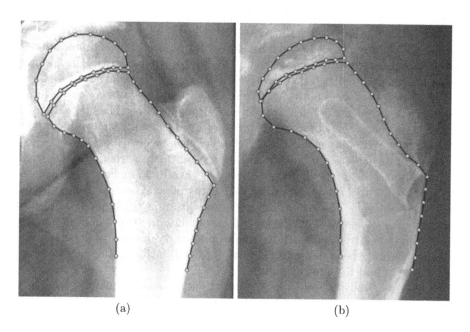

(a)                                                                (b)

**Fig. 1.** An example of 58 points annotated on (a) a healthy child hip and (b) a hip affected by Perthes disease. Note that the landmark points were placed automatically using a Random Forest Regression-Voting system (see Sect. 3.3 for details).

There are only very few methods that utilise computer vision to analyse and study Perthes disease and, to the best of our knowledge, so far no computer vision based methods have been presented to classify between Perthes hips and healthy hips. A semi-automatic radiograph-based method was created for the quantitative analysis of the hips of children with Perthes [11], where manual landmark points initialised the femoral head contour, and a gradient operator with linear interpolation was used for the final contour location. The bone loss in the affected hip was identified by comparing the area included in the affected contour with that in the contour of the contra-lateral unaffected hip using the brightness of pixels (from 0 to 255 grey levels).

Chan et al. [12] used statistical shape modelling to understand the morphological deformities in both Perthes disease and slipped capital femoral epiphysis (SCFE) using 3D CT scans. Their results showed that the analysis of femoral shape during growth and in various disease stages are contributing to the understanding of normal and abnormal hip shape deviations, the latter of which may affect the risk of developing hip osteoarthritis.

Currently, in clinical practice, any method to diagnose or classify stages of Perthes disease or to determine patient outcomes are done manually by the treating surgeon.

In this study, we investigate how the radiographic shape, texture and appearance of children's hips can be used to distinguish children's hips affected by Perthes disease from healthy children's hips. Our analysis is based on outlining the proximal femur with landmark points and applying statistical shape and appearance modelling [13,14]. We test each of the three parameter sets (shape, texture, and appearance) individually to identify if any one of them outperforms the others as a classification feature. We use a Random Forest classifier (RF) [15] for this task, comparing our automatically obtained classification results to data manually categorised by clinicians (Perthes vs. healthy hips).

Further, we investigate the classification performance when the landmark point positions are obtained fully automatically via a Random Forest Regression-Voting (RFRV) [16,17] system, rather than using manual landmark annotations (i.e. point positions). The latter are very time-consuming to obtain and prone to inconsistencies. Therefore, creating a fully automatic method to both annotate the hip and classify disease status would greatly reduce the amount of time clinicians need to spend analysing patient data, and facilitate the integration of such a system into the clinical workflow.

Finally, we analyse how classification results based on manual landmark annotations compare to classification results based on fully automatically obtained landmark annotations. Our results demonstrate that our fully automatic classification system is able to replicate the healthy vs Perthes classification by clinicians, with an area under the ROC curve (AUC) of 98%.

## 2   Background

Locating landmarks on medical images is an important first step in many musculoskeletal analysis tasks, particularly those requiring geometric measurements of the shape of structures (see Fig. 1 for a landmark annotation example). Many methods have been proposed for automating landmark localisation, with some of the most effective using Random Forest Regression-Voting (RFRV) [16,17] which has been used for automatically locating landmarks along the proximal femur in radiographs of adult hips [16].

Techniques for analysing human skeletal structures [18] and their associated diseases are well established in describing the differences between healthy and diseased bone. Waarsing et al. [19] constructed statistical shape and appearance models for the left and right proximal femurs for cases of osteoarthritis. Their results show that subtle shape and appearance changes can be identified with these models in cases where traditional clinical measures might miss them. Whitmarsh et al. [20] used statistical shape and appearance models to distinguish fractured bones from a non-fractured control group using Fisher Linear Discriminant Analysis. They concluded that the proposed model-based fracture risk estimation method may improve upon the current standard in clinical practice.

**Table 1.** A breakdown of the Perthes and healthy radiograph dataset with the total numbers of annotated and unannotated images.

|         | Annotated | Unannotated | Total |
|---------|-----------|-------------|-------|
| Healthy | 1109      | 284         | 1393  |
| Perthes | 70        | 317         | 387   |
| Total   | 1179      | 601         | 1780  |

Thomson et al. [21] analysed the shape and texture of the tibia in radiographs of osteoarthritis-affected knees using Random Forests for classification. Their fully automatic system achieved an AUC of 0.849 when combining both radiographic shape and texture, up from 0.789 when using shape alone. Their results demonstrate the effectiveness of using both radiographic shape and texture for classification.

Radiographic shape and appearance have also been used to estimate bone age [22] from radiographs of children's hands using a RFRV system. The method achieved mean absolute prediction errors of 0.57 years and 0.58 years for females and males, respectively.

## 3   Method

### 3.1   Data Collection and Annotation

The dataset consists of (a) 387 AP pelvic radiographs of children (aged between 2–11 years) affected by Perthes and (b) 1393 radiographs of children not affected by Perthes (aged between 2–11 years). 1109 of the healthy cases, and 70 of the diseased cases were manually annotated with 58 points as shown in Fig. 1. There were no manual annotations for the remainder of the images. For the sake of convenience, the annotated dataset and unannotated dataset will henceforth be referred to by "Data-A" and "Data-U", respectively. See Table 1 for a breakdown of the total number of radiographs.

This dataset is very challenging due to the natural growth stage during childhood, meaning the femur has growth areas such as the femoral head and greater trochanter. In addition, Perthes disease can have a significant effect on radiographic shape and appearance. Figure 2 shows some examples of the challenging nature of the dataset. Even clinicians consider the task of manually annotating these hips (to create a ground truth) difficult, which increases the complexity of developing a system that would do this automatically.

### 3.2   Shape and Appearance Modelling

A statistical shape model (SSM) consists of a linear model of the distribution of a set of landmarks across a set of images. In the following we provide a brief summary on how to generate an SSM, for more details see [13]. To generate

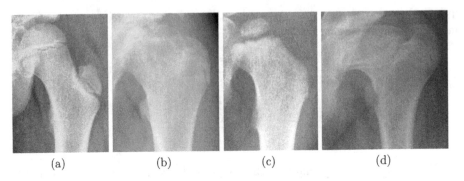

(a)        (b)        (c)        (d)

**Fig. 2.** Examples of healthy hips: (a) shows an older child but with visible growth plates on the femoral head and greater trochanter, and (b) is a 2 year old child with an early growth stage femoral head. Examples of Perthes hips: (c) demonstrates the difficulty of identifying the outline of the superior femoral head in some cases, and (d) gives an example of the extreme deformities of the femoral head.

an SSM, the training data is a set of $n$ images $\mathbf{I}$ with annotations $\mathbf{x}_l$ of a set of $N$ landmark points $l = 1, \ldots, N$ on each image. In this study, we use both manually obtained landmark positions and automatically obtained landmark positions. To begin, each image is aligned to a standard reference frame using a similarity transformation $T$ with parameters $\theta$. An SSM can then be created by applying principal component analysis (PCA) to all $n$ training shapes in the reference frame, generating a linear model of shape variation that describes the position of each point $l$ by

$$\mathbf{x}_l = T_\theta(\bar{\mathbf{x}}_l + \mathbf{P}_{sl}\mathbf{b}_s) \tag{1}$$

where $\bar{\mathbf{x}}_l$ is the mean position of the landmark point in the reference frame, $\mathbf{P}_{sl}$ is a set of modes of shape variation relating to the landmark point, and $\mathbf{b}_s$ are the shape model parameters.

Using dimensionality reduction, SSMs can be used to provide a compact quantitative description of the shape of the bone, which is very useful for classification tasks. However, SSMs only consider the distribution of the landmark point positions and hence only describe the radiographic shape of the bone. Perthes disease is known for avascular necrosis of the femoral head, which in radiographs shows as opposite pixel intensities compared to healthy bone. Statistical appearance models (SAMs), as used in the well-known Active Appearance Models [14] method, apply PCA-based linear modelling to both landmark point positions (i.e. shape) and pixel intensities (i.e. texture).

In the following we provide a brief summary on how to generate an SAM, for more details see [14]. To build a texture model, a patch comprising the set of landmark points is sampled from each training image. All patches are shape-normalised and texture-normalised to generate shape-free patches where global lightning variations have been removed. Each patch is then sampled into a texture vector $\mathbf{g}$ representing the texture of a particular training image in the reference frame. Given the set of $n$ normalised texture vectors, PCA can be applied to generate a linear texture model

$$\mathbf{g} = \bar{\mathbf{g}} + \mathbf{P}_g \mathbf{b}_g \quad and \quad \mathbf{b}_g = \mathbf{P}_g^T (\mathbf{g} - \bar{\mathbf{g}}) \tag{2}$$

where $\bar{\mathbf{g}}$ is the mean texture, $\mathbf{P}_g$ are the modes of texture variation, and $\mathbf{b}_g$ are the texture model parameters.

SAMs combine both shape and texture models to also capture correlations between shape and texture. Following the description above, the appearance of an image can be summarised using shape parameters $\mathbf{b}_s$ and texture parameters $\mathbf{b}_g$. To generate an SAM, appearance vector $\mathbf{b}$ can be defined by

$$\mathbf{b} = \begin{pmatrix} \mathbf{W}_s \mathbf{b}_s \\ \mathbf{b}_g \end{pmatrix} \tag{3}$$

where $\mathbf{W}_s$ is a diagonal matrix of weights to account for the difference in units between the shape and texture models (e.g. coordinates vs pixel intensities). Applying PCA to $\mathbf{b}$ yields an SAM given by

$$\mathbf{b} = \mathbf{P}_c \mathbf{c} \tag{4}$$

where $\mathbf{P}_c$ is a set of modes of appearance variation, and $\mathbf{c}$ are the appearance model parameters. Applying SSMs and SAMs to radiographic images provides a meaningful way to capture the variation in radiographic shape and texture that may allow to distinguish between proximal femurs affected by Perthes disease and healthy proximal femurs. In this study, we explore the effectiveness of using (i) shape model parameters $\mathbf{b}_s$; (ii) texture model parameters $\mathbf{b}_g$; or (iii) appearance model parameters $\mathbf{c}$ for classifying diseased and healthy hips.

### 3.3   Automatic Landmark Annotation

In light of applying the proposed technology in clinical practice it would be necessary for the system to be fully automatic. That is, the proposed classification system would need to be able to automatically place the 58 landmark points. For this purpose, we trained a RFRV system as presented in [16,17]. We used Data-A as training data for the system and performed five-fold cross-validation experiments (i.e. the data was randomly split into five even blocks and each block was used once for testing with the remaining blocks used for training). To be able to estimate the performance of a fully automatic classification system and compare this to a classification system based on manual ground truth, we combined the test results of all five folds to obtain a set of automatic annotations for Data-A. Note that because we used five-fold cross-validation experiments to generate the automatic annotations for Data-A, all automatic landmark point positions were obtained without training and testing on the same data. Comparing the manual and automatic landmark annotations for Data-A shows that the RFRV system achieved a point-to-curve-error of 4% of the femoral shaft width for 95% of all 1179 images and a median accuracy of less than 1.8% of the femoral shaft width.

Furthermore, the majority of our Perthes data (317 images) are unannotated. To allow us to utilise this data, Data-U, for evaluating the classification performance in this study, we randomly chose one of the five cross-validation RFRV systems trained on Data-A and used this to fully automatically annotate all images in Data-U.

## 4    Evaluation

To classify between Perthes and healthy hips, we obtained the shape, texture and appearance model parameter values based on annotated (manually and/or automatically) proximal femurs (healthy and Perthes) as shown in Fig. 1. We used the shape, texture and appearance model parameter values as classification features. Throughout the classification evaluation, we performed 5-fold cross-validation experiments (i.e. the data was randomly split into five even blocks and each block was used once for testing with the remaining blocks used for training) and we report the average classification performance over all five runs.

For all classification experiments, we used Random Forests (RF) [15] with 500 trees as the classifier. We applied bootstrapping, and the number of features to consider for each node split was set to $\sqrt{n\_features}$ with $n\_features$ being the number of shape, texture or appearance model parameter values. When obtaining the shape, texture and appearance model parameter values, we constrained the number of modes of variation such that the texture model explained 85% and the shape/appearance models each explained 98% of the data variation. We report the results using receiver operator characteristic (ROC) curves that show the true positive rate (TPR) against the false positive rate (FPR), along with the area under the curve (AUC).

### 4.1    Data-A Perthes Classification

Data-A includes manual annotations for 70 Perthes and 1109 healthy images. The classification results based on the model parameters obtained from the manual annotations (see Fig. 3) show that texture does not perform as well as shape or appearance. The best classification results were obtained when using the shape or appearance model parameter values with an AUC of 0.93 (SD: ±0.06) and 0.93 (SD: ±0.03) respectively.

### 4.2    Balanced Data-A Perthes Classification

Data-A has an imbalance between classes (70 Perthes cases vs. 1109 healthy cases) which could be a disadvantage in the above experiments. To investigate the impact of this class imbalance on performance, we took a random subset of 100 healthy hips from Data-A such that the classes were much closer in number, and re-ran the classification experiments. Figure 4 shows that this leads to improved classification results for all models, significantly boosting the texture model classification performance with an AUC of 0.96 (SD: ±0.02).

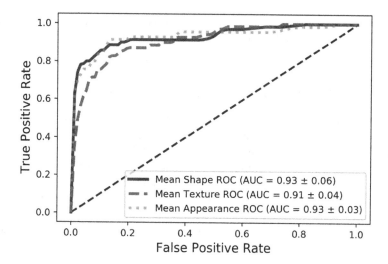

**Fig. 3.** Cross-validation ROC curves for Perthes-healthy classification when using shape, texture or appearance parameters based on Data-A (70 Perthes and 1109 healthy). All results were obtained using manual ground truth landmark annotations.

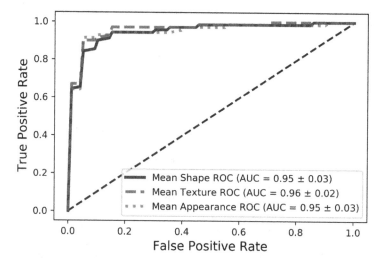

**Fig. 4.** Cross-validation ROC curves for Perthes-healthy classification when using shape, texture or appearance parameters based on a subset of Data-A with a more balanced number of healthy and Perthes data (70 Perthes and 100 healthy). All results were obtained using manual ground truth landmark annotations.

Training the classifier on a proportionally large amount of normal, healthy hips can create a bias towards the radiographic shape and appearance of healthy hips. Due to the effects of disease, Perthes cases show a much wider variation in the radiographic shape, texture and appearance parameter values. It may, thus, be beneficial to keep the datasets as balanced as possible. The results in Fig. 4 demonstrate the potential performance improvements when using a balanced dataset.

### 4.3    Fully Automatic Shape and Appearance Analysis

Our fully automatic system uses RFRV to locate the landmark points without the need for any manual intervention. Figure 5 shows the fully automatically obtained classification results for Data-U (284 healthy and 317 Perthes) where the model parameter values were obtained from the automatically located landmark points. The best performance was achieved when using the shape or appearance model parameters with an AUC of 0.98 (SD: ± 0.01). Overall, the classification results for Data-U (using automatic landmark annotations) are better than the results obtained for Data-A (using manual landmark annotations).

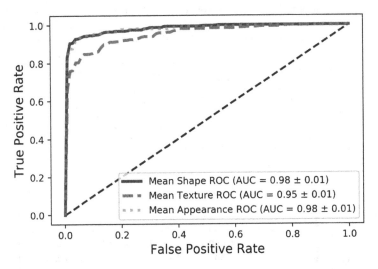

**Fig. 5.** Cross-validation ROC curves for the fully automatically obtained classification results for Data-U when using shape, texture or appearance model parameters. All landmark point positions were obtained automatically using the developed RFRV system.

Similar to the manual annotation results, the shape and appearance parameters outperform the texture parameters in the fully automatic analysis. It is noteworthy that Data-U contains many more Perthes cases than Data-A. Therefore, this setting is a more challenging task due to the increased range of radiographic shape and appearance variations across Perthes cases. This is in particular the case because the RFRV system used to automatically locate the landmark points in Data-U was trained using Data-A which only includes 70 Perthes cases in total.

## 4.4 Manual Versus Automatic Classification

The automatic classification results for Data-U show an improvement in performance over the manual classification results for Data-A. However, this improvement in performance may originate from the difference in datasets. To directly compare the fully automatic classification performance to a classification system based on manual landmark annotations, we re-ran the classification experiments for Data-A using the automatically obtained Data-A landmark annotations (see Sect. 3.3) rather than the manual ground truth Data-A annotations.

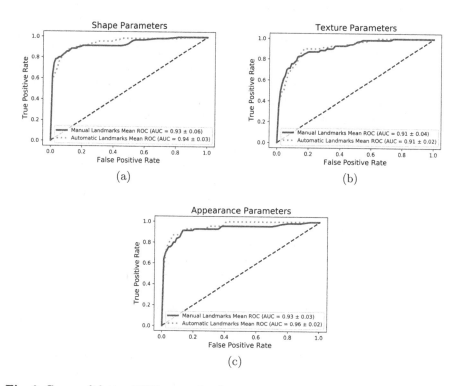

**Fig. 6.** Cross-validation ROC curves for the comparison between the manual and automatic classification results for Data-A when using (a) shape, (b) texture and (c) appearance model parameters.

Figure 6 gives the results of the comparison for each of the parameter sets. The results show that the fully automatic classification system performs better than the classification system based on manual landmark annotations. The best performance was obtained when using the appearance model parameters with AUCs of 0.96 (SD: $\pm 0.02$) and 0.93 (SD: $\pm 0.03$) for the automatic and manual systems, respectively. These results demonstrate that we are able to fully automatically annotate diseased and healthy hips, and accurately classify the data, even when the data is imbalanced.

# 5  Discussion and Conclusions

We have evaluated a radiograph-based classification system to distinguish proximal femurs affected by Perthes disease from healthy ones by using shape, texture and appearance model parameters. We have investigated how each set of parameters performs using a Random Forest classifier to identify healthy and Perthes hips. Our experiments show that the combination of shape and texture (appearance) performs best, achieving an AUC of 98% when using a fully automatic classification system.

In all our experiments, except for the balanced dataset experiments, classification based on shape model parameters outperformed the classification based on texture model parameters. Although the radiographic texture of the proximal femur may be affected by the radiolucency effect (caused by the dying bone of the femoral head in the early-mid stages of Perthes [9]), changes in bone shape seem to be more discriminative. This highlights the impact of Perthes disease on the (radiographic) shape of the proximal femur. However, the discriminatory power of texture may improve when using a balanced dataset.

Our comparison of the performance of a fully automatic classification system to a classification system based on manual landmark annotations demonstrates that improved performance can be achieved when using automatically identified landmark positions. A possible explanation for this is that the automatic annotations are placed more consistently, reducing random errors introduced by manual landmark annotations.

We have shown a viable system based on statistical shape and appearance models to automatically classify whether a hip is affected by Perthes disease or not. The proposed system would save clinicians' time, and produce accurate and robust results in clinical practice. In addition, such a system would be of benefit to support less experienced clinicians' or in a non-specialty clinical setting.

Further work will add more manually annotated diseased data during training for the comparison of the agreement between clinical diagnosis (Perthes vs. healthy hips) and the outputs of the automatic system. As Perthes is a rare disease, the availability of Perthes data compared to healthy data is low. Future work will focus on utilising a balanced dataset with as many Perthes cases as possible for developing (i.e. training) an automatic classification system, and then evaluating the system on an unseen imbalanced dataset to reflect the data availability in clinical practice.

Moreover, the system could be extended to use radiographic shape and appearance in combination with clinical data to also classify (i) the stage of disease progression [5,6]; (ii) prognostic outcomes [7–9]; and (iii) long term patients' outcomes [10]. Once we have collected more data, we will also be able to explore outcomes based on different age groups which is important because younger ages, for example, have a higher chance of the hip restoring to relative normality.

**Acknowledgements.** A. K. Davison was funded by Arthritis Research UK as part of the ORCHiD project. C. Lindner was funded by the Engineering and Physical Sciences Research Council, UK (EP/M012611/1) and by the Medical Research Council, UK (MR/S00405X/1). Manual landmark annotations were provided by the Medical Student Annotation Collaborative (Grace Airey, Evan Araia, Aishwarya Avula, Emily Gargan, Mihika Joshi, Muhammad Khan, Kantida Koysombat, Jason Lee, Sophie Munday, and Allen Roby).

# References

1. Perry, D.C.: The epidemiology and etiology of Perthes' disease. In: Koo, K.-H., Mont, M.A., Jones, L.C. (eds.) Osteonecrosis, pp. 419–425. Springer, Heidelberg (2014). https://doi.org/10.1007/978-3-642-35767-1_58
2. Hall, A., Barker, D.: The age distribution of Legg-Perthes disease: an analysis using Sartwell's incubation period model. Am. J. Epidemiol. **120**(4), 531–536 (1984)
3. Wiig, O., Terjesen, T., Svenningsen, S., Lie, S.: The epidemiology and aetiology of Perthes disease in Norway: a nationwide study of 425 patients. J. Bone Joint Surg. Br. **88**(9), 1217–1223 (2006). https://doi.org/10.1302/0301-620X.88B9.17400
4. Hunter, J.: (iv) Legg Calvé Perthes' disease. Curr. Orthop. **18**(4), 273–283 (2004). https://doi.org/10.1016/j.cuor.2004.06.001
5. Waldenstrom, H.: The first stages of coxa plana. Acta Orthop. Scand. **5**(1–4), 1–34 (1934)
6. Joseph, B.: Natural history of early onset and late-onset Legg-Calve-Perthes disease. J. Pediatr. Orthop. **31**(Suppl. 2), S152–S155 (2011). https://doi.org/10.1097/BPO.0b013e318223b423
7. Catterall, A.: Natural history, classification, and x-ray signs in Legg-Calvé-Perthes' disease. Acta Orthop. Belg. **46**(4), 346–351 (1980)
8. Salter, R., Thompson, G.: Legg-Calvé-Perthes disease: the prognostic significance of the subchondral fracture and a two-group classification of the femoral head involvement. J. Bone Joint Surg. Am. **66**(4), 479–489 (1984)
9. Herring, J., Neustadt, J., Williams, J., Early, J., Browne, R.: The lateral pillar classification of Legg-Calvé-Perthes disease. J. Pediatr. Orthop. **12**(2), 143–150 (1992)
10. Stulberg, S., Cooperman, D., Wallensten, R.: The natural history of Legg-Calvé-Perthes disease. J. Bone Joint Surg. Am. **763**(7), 1095–1108 (1981)
11. Mouravliansky, N., Matsopoulos, G., Nikita, K., Uzunoglu, N., Pistevos, G.: An image processing technique for the quantitative analysis of hip disorder in Perthes' disease. In: Proceedings of 18th Annual International Conference of the IEEE Engineering in Medicine and Biology Society - EMBC 1996, vol. 3, pp. 1103–1104. IEEE (1996). https://doi.org/10.1109/IEMBS.1996.652728
12. Chan, E., Farnsworth, C., Koziol, J., Hosalkar, H., Sah, R.: Statistical shape modeling of proximal femoral shape deformities in Legg-Calvé-Perthes disease and slipped capital femoral epiphysis. Osteoarthritis Cartilage **31**(3), 443–449 (2013). https://doi.org/10.1016/j.joca.2012.12.007
13. Cootes, T., Taylor, C., Cooper, D., Graham, J.: Active shape models - their training and application. Comput. Vis. Image Understand. **61**(1), 38–59 (1995). https://doi.org/10.1006/cviu.1995.1004
14. Cootes, T., Edwards, G., Taylor, C.: Active appearance models. IEEE Trans. Pattern Anal. Mach. Intell. **23**(6), 681–685 (2001). https://doi.org/10.1109/34.927467

15. Breiman, L.: Random forests. Mach. Learn. **45**(1), 5–32 (2001). https://doi.org/10.1023/A:1010933404324

16. Lindner, C., Thiagarajah, S., Wilkinson, J., The arcOGEN Consortium, Wallis, G., Cootes, T.: Fully automatic segmentation of the proximal femur using random forest regression voting. IEEE Trans. Med. Imaging **32**(8), 1462–1472 (2013), https://doi.org/10.1109/TMI.2013.2258030

17. Lindner, C., Bromiley, P., Ionita, M., Cootes, T.: Robust and accurate shape model matching using random forest regression-voting. IEEE Trans. Pattern Anal. Mach. Intell. **37**(9), 1862–1874 (2015). https://doi.org/10.1109/TPAMI.2014.2382106

18. Sarkalkan, N., Weinans, H., Zadpoor, A.: Statistical shape and appearance models of bones. Bone **60**, 129–140 (2014). https://doi.org/10.1016/j.bone.2013.12.006

19. Waarsing, J., Rozendaal, R., Verhaar, J., Bierma-Zeinstra, S., Weinans, H.: A statistical model of shape and density of the proximal femur in relation to radiological and clinical OA of the hip. Osteoarthritis Cartilage **18**(6), 787–794 (2010). https://doi.org/10.1016/j.joca.2010.02.003

20. Whitmarsh, T., et al.: A statistical model of shape and bone mineral density distribution of the proximal femur for fracture risk assessment. In: Fichtinger, G., Martel, A., Peters, T. (eds.) MICCAI 2011. LNCS, vol. 6892, pp. 393–400. Springer, Heidelberg (2011). https://doi.org/10.1007/978-3-642-23629-7_48

21. Thomson, J., O'Neill, T., Felson, D., Cootes, T.: Automated shape and texture analysis for detection of osteoarthritis from radiographs of the knee. In: Navab, N., Hornegger, J., Wells, W.M., Frangi, A.F. (eds.) MICCAI 2015. LNCS, vol. 9350, pp. 127–134. Springer, Cham (2015). https://doi.org/10.1007/978-3-319-24571-3_16

22. Adeshina, S., Cootes, T., Adams, J.: Automatic assessment of bone age using statistical models of appearance and random forest regression voting. In: Proceedings of 13th International Conference on Electronics, Computer and Computation - ICECCO, pp. 1–6. IEEE (2017). https://doi.org/10.1109/ICECCO.2017.8333314

# Deep Learning Based Rib Centerline Extraction and Labeling

Matthias Lenga$^{(\boxtimes)}$, Tobias Klinder, Christian Bürger, Jens von Berg,
Astrid Franz, and Cristian Lorenz

Philips Research Europe, Hamburg, Germany
matthias.lenga@philips.com

**Abstract.** Automated extraction and labeling of rib centerlines is a typically needed prerequisite for more advanced assisted reading tools that help the radiologist to efficiently inspect all 24 ribs in a computed tomography (CT) volume. In this paper, we combine a deep learning-based rib detection with a dedicated centerline extraction algorithm applied to the detection result for the purpose of fast, robust and accurate rib centerline extraction and labeling from CT volumes. More specifically, we first apply a fully convolutional neural network to generate a probability map for detecting the *first rib* pair, the *twelfth rib* pair, and the collection of all *intermediate ribs*. In a second stage, a newly designed centerline extraction algorithm is applied to this multi-label probability map. Finally, the distinct detection of first and twelfth rib separately, allows to derive individual rib labels by simple sorting and counting the detected centerlines. We applied our method to CT volumes with an isotropic voxel spacing of 1.5 mm from 113 patients which included a variety of different challenges and achieved a mean centerline accuracy of 0.723 mm with respect to manual centerline annotations. The presented approach can be applied to similar tracing problems, such as detecting the spinal column centerline.

**Keywords:** Rib segmentation · Centerline tracing · Deep learning
Fully convolutional neural networks · Whole-body CT scans · Trauma

## 1 Introduction

The reading of the ribs from three-dimensional (3D) computed tomography (CT) scans is a typical task in radiology, e.g. to find bone lesions or identify fractures. During reading, each of the 24 ribs needs to be followed individually while scrolling through the slices. As a result, this task is time-consuming and rib abnormalities are likely to be overlooked.

In order to assist reading, efficient visualization schemes or methods for navigation support are required. These applications are typically based on the rib centerlines [1,2]. Despite their generally high contrast, automated extraction of

© Springer Nature Switzerland AG 2019
T. Vrtovec et al. (Eds.): MSKI 2018, LNCS 11404, pp. 99–113, 2019.
https://doi.org/10.1007/978-3-030-11166-3_9

the rib centerlines from CT is challenging. For example, image noise and artifacts impede the extraction, but also other bony structures in close vicinity (most prominently the vertebra), as well as severe pathologies. Finally, anatomical labeling of the extracted centerlines (i.e. knowing which one for example is the "7th right rib") is usually desirable. From an algorithmic perspective, this task is trivial if all 24 ribs are correctly extracted, as simply counting left and right ribs from cranial to caudal would be sufficient. Obviously, this task becomes significantly more challenging once the rib-cage is only partially imaged or once a rib is missing (e.g. due to pathologies or missed detection in a previous step).

A wide range of different approaches has been proposed in the past for rib centerline extraction partially also including their labeling. Tracing based approaches, as in [3,4] aim at iteratively following the ribs. As such approaches rely on an initial seed point detection per rib, an entire rib is easily missed once a corresponding seed point was not detected. Alternatively, potential rib candidates can be first detected in the entire volume which then need to be grouped to obtain ribs, as for example done in [5]. However, the removal of other falsely detected structures remains a crucial task. Attempts have been made to additionally integrate prior knowledge by means of geometrical rib cage centerline models [2,6]. Nevertheless, such approaches may struggle with deviations from the model in terms of pathologies.

In this paper, we propose a two-stage approach combining deep learning and classic image processing techniques to overcome several of the limitations listed above. Rib probability maps are calculated at first using a fully convolutional neural network (FCNN) (Sect. 2.2), and then the centerlines are reconstructed using a specifically designed centerline extraction algorithm (Sect. 2.3). In particular, three distinct rib probability maps are calculated (*first rib*, *twelfth rib* or *intermediate rib*). By knowing the first and/or twelfth rib, labeling can be solved easily by iterative counting. This scheme also works in case of partial rib cages (for example if only the upper or lower part is shown). Evaluation is carried out on a representative number of 113 cases.

## 2   Methods

### 2.1   Data

Our data set consists in total of 113 image volumes containing 59 thorax as well as 54 full body CT scans. The data includes a wide range of typical challenges, such as variation in the field of view leading to partly visible or missing ribs (3 patients with first rib missing, 38 patients with at least partially missing twelfth rib), various types of rib fractures, spine scoliosis (14 patients) strong contrast-uptake around the first rib (33 patients), implants in other bony structures (7 around the sternum, 2 around the spine, and 2 around the femur/humerus), several different devices with similar intensity to the ribs such as catheters or cables (57 patients).

In each image, we annotated rib centerlines by manually placing spline control points. The rib centerlines were then obtained using cubic spline interpolation.

For each image volume, we generated a label mask by dilating the corresponding centerlines with a radius of 3.0 mm. Four different labels are assigned to the classes *background*, *first rib*, *twelfth rib* and *intermediate rib*.

## 2.2 Multi-label Rib Probability Map Generation

For rib detection, we first apply a FCNN in order to generate probability maps which are subsequently fed into the tracing algorithm (Sect. 2.3). More specifically, we formulate our task as a four-class problem, where the network yields for each voxel $v_{ijk}$ of the volume a four-dimensional vector $p_{ijk} \in [0,1]^4$. The components $p_{ijk,0}, p_{ijk,1}, p_{ijk,2}, p_{ijk,3}$ can be interpreted as probabilities that the associated voxel belongs to the classes *background*, *first rib (pair)*, *twelfth rib (pair)* or *intermediate rib (pairs)*, respectively. Distinct classes for the first and the twelfth rib were introduced to deal with differences in anatomy (especially for the first rib) while significantly simplifying the following labeling procedure. By using the relative to location of the intermediate ribs to the first and twelfth rib, labeling of the ribs can be achieved efficiently. Moreover, knowing the potential location of first or twelfth rib enables labeling even in cases of partial rib cages. Details are provided in Sect. 2.3 below. We favored the parsimonious four-class learning task over training a neural network for detecting each individual rib, resulting in a 25-class (24 ribs plus background) classification problem, due to several reasons: (a) The four-class network in combination with our iterative tracing approach seems sufficient for robustly solving the problem at hand, (b) due to the similar appearance of intermediate ribs, we do not expect the 25-class network to be able to identify internal ribs reliably, (c) the 25-class approach would cause a higher memory footprint and runtime during training and inference.

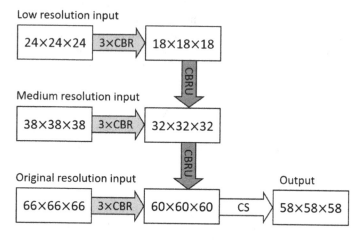

**Fig. 1.** Foveal architecture with three resolution levels. The feature extraction pathways (green), consisting of three CBR blocks, are integrated using CBRU blocks (blue). The final CS block consists of a $3 \times 3 \times 3$ valid convolution and a soft-max layer. (Color figure online)

**Table 1.** Input configuration of the network layers.

|  | Input patch size (voxel) | Patch voxel spacing (mm) |
|---|---|---|
| $L_H$ original resolution | $66 \times 66 \times 66$ | $1.5 \times 1.5 \times 1.5$ |
| $L_M$ medium resolution | $38 \times 38 \times 38$ | $3.0 \times 3.0 \times 3.0$ |
| $L_L$ low resolution | $24 \times 24 \times 24$ | $6.0 \times 6.0 \times 6.0$ |

As network architecture, we chose the Foveal network described in [7]. Basically, the network is composed of two different types of layer modules, CBR and CBRU blocks (Fig. 1). A CBR block consists of a $3 \times 3 \times 3$ valid convolution (C) followed by batch normalization (B) and a rectified linear unit activation (R). A CBRU block is a CBR block followed by an average unpooling layer (U). Since we favor fast network execution times and a moderate GPU memory consumption, we decided to use three resolution layers $L_H, L_M, L_L$, each composed of three CBR blocks. Differently sized image patches with different isotropic voxel spacings are fed into the layers as input (Table 1). The low and medium resolution pathways $L_L, L_M$ are integrated into the high resolution layer $L_H$ using CBRU blocks. Implementation details and further remarks concerning the architecture performance can be found in [7].

As preprocessing, the CT images are resampled to an isotropic spacing of 1.5 mm using linear interpolation. For image normalization we used intensity window normalization with an intensity window of [500, 2000] HU and clipping at the window boundaries. The network was trained by minimizing the cross entropy on mini-batches containing 8 patches (each at three different resolutions) drawn from eight randomly selected images. In order to compensate for the class imbalance between background and rib voxels, we used the following randomized sampling strategy: 10% of the patch centers were sampled from the bounding box of the first rib pair, 10% from the bounding box of the twelfth rib pair and 30% from the bounding box of the intermediate ribs. The remaining 50% patch centers were uniformly sampled from the entire volume. As an update rule, we chose AdaDelta [8] in combination with a learning rate schedule. For data augmentation, the patches were randomly scaled and rotated around all three axes. The neural network was implemented with CNTK version 2.2 and trained for 1200 epochs on a GeForce GTX 1080. The network training could be completed within a few hours and network inference times were ranging from approximately 5 to 20 s, depending on the size of the input CT volume.

## 2.3   Centerline Extraction and Labeling

In order to robustly obtain rib centerlines, we designed an algorithm that specifically incorporates the available information from the multi-label probability map. It basically consists of four distinct steps:

1. Determination of a rib-cage bounding box.
2. Detection of an initial left and right rib.
3. Tracing of the detected ribs and detecting neighboring ribs.
4. Rib labeling.

Steps 1 to 3 are performed on the *combined probability map*, adding the results of the three non-background classes and limiting the sum to a total probability of 1.0, i.e. to each voxel $v_{ijk}$ we assign the value $q_{ijk} := \min\{p_{ijk,1}+p_{ijk,2}+p_{ijk,3}, 1\}$.

**Step 1: Bounding Box Detection.** Generally, the given CT volume is assumed to cover at least a large portion of the rib cage, but may extend beyond it. Therefore, we first determine a search region in order to identify the visible ribs. Based on the axial image slices, a two-dimensional (2D) bounding rectangle is computed using a probability threshold of 0.5 on the combined probability map. To suppress spurious responses, we require a minimal 2D box of size 30 mm × 10 mm to be a *valid* bounding box. From the set of valid 2D bounding boxes, a 3D bounding box is calculated from the largest connected stack in vertical direction. The 3D bounding box is strictly speaking not a box, but has inclined faces. Each of the four faces results from a linear regression of the slice wise determined four border positions, having the advantage of being robust against outliers and being able to represent to some extent the narrowing of the rib cage from abdomen to shoulders (Fig. 2(a) and (b)).

**Step 2: Initial Rib Detection.** From the approximate rib cage bounding box obtained in Step 1, we derive an initial cross-sectional search window to detect the ribs. For that purpose, anchor point $a_l, a_r$ are chosen at 25% and 75% of the left-to-right extension of the box section at medium axial level. Then sagittal 2D search regions centered at $a_l$ and $a_r$ of spacial extension 100 mm × 100 mm are defined (Fig. 2(a) and (b)). In each of these regions an initialization point exceeding a probability of 0.5 is determined. We remark that this point may be located at the rib border. To locate the rib center, we sample the probability values in a spherical region of 15 mm diameter around the initialization point. Next, the probability weighted center of mass $c_0 \in \mathbb{R}^3$ and the probability weighted covariance matrix $\Sigma_0 \in \mathbb{R}^{3\times3}$ of the voxel coordinates are calculated. Finally, we use $c_0$ as rib center estimate and the eigenvector $t_0 \in \mathbb{R}^3$ corresponding to the largest eigenvalue of $\Sigma_0$ as estimation of the tangential direction. The position $c_0$ is added to the list of rib center line control points.

**Step 3: Rib Tracing and Detection of Neighboring Ribs.** Based on the initial rib detection result from Step 2, the rib response in the probability map is traced in an iterated scheme ($i = 0, 1, 2, \ldots$) consisting of the following three actions:

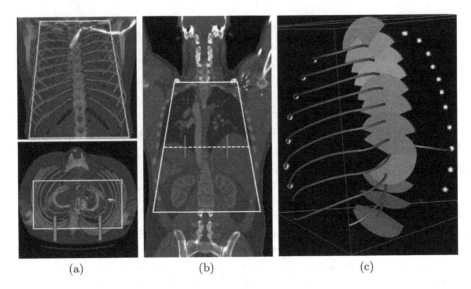

       (a)                (b)              (c)

**Fig. 2.** (a) Neural network output (green: first rib; red: intermediate rib; blue: twelfth rib) and approximate three-dimensional (3D) bounding box of the rib cage (yellow) in coronal (top) and axial view (bottom). The lower image depicts in light blue the two search regions for rib detection. (b) Schematic representation of the vertical stack of two-dimensional bounding boxes (red) in coronal view and the approximate 3D bounding box of the rib cage resulting from the largest connected stack in vertical direction by linear regression (yellow). The dashed yellow line marks the box section at medium axial level. The two search regions used for initial rib detection are depicted in light blue. (c) Traced ribs (red) are shown on top of a sagittal cross-section of the probability map. The fan-like search regions for neighboring ribs are depicted in yellow. (Color figure online)

(a) Starting from $c_i$ move in tangential direction $t_i$ until a voxel with combined probability value $q_{ijk} < 0.5$ is encountered or a maximal moving distance of 7.5 mm is reached.

(b) Calculate the weighted mean vector $c_{i+1} \in \mathbb{R}^3$ in a spherical region around the current position. Add $c_{i+1}$ to the list of rib center line control points and move to $c_{i+1}$.

(c) Calculate the probability weighted covariance matrix $\Sigma_{i+1} \in \mathbb{R}^{3\times3}$ in a spherical region around $c_{i+1}$ and compute the tangential direction $t_{i+1} \in \mathbb{R}^3$, see Step 2.

This scheme is iterated until the moving distance in the current iteration falls below a predefined threshold of 3.0 mm. In that case, a forward-looking mechanism is triggered which aims at bridging local drop-outs of the probability response. More precisely, the algorithm searches for a voxel with a combined

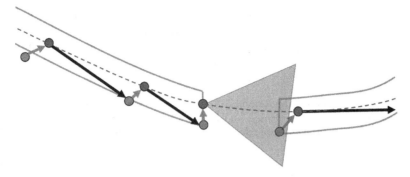

**Fig. 3.** Schematic representation of the iterative tracing algorithm. Each red point corresponds to a probability weighted mean vector $c_i$ in the spherical region around the associated preceding position which is depicted by a yellow point connected by a yellow arrow (see Step 3, b). The black arrows correspond to a movement in tangential direction $t_i$ (see Step 3, a). The blue triangle depicts the cone-shaped search region used by the forward-looking mechanism. The rib center line resulting from a spline interpolation of the control points $c_i$ is depicted by the dashed red line. (Color figure online)

probability value exceeding 0.5 within a cone-shaped region. This voxel then serves as continuation point for the iterative tracing procedure described above (Fig. 3).

Tracing from the initial starting point $c_0$ is performed in both possible directions and results are finally concatenated which yields a centerline of the full rib represented by the point sequence $\{c_0, c_1, \dots\}$. After the tracing of one rib is completed, the resulting centerline is inserted into the list of rib centerlines $L$ which is ordered in vertical direction from feet to head.

This collection is extended in a step wise fashion by detecting adjacent so far untraced ribs using fan-like 2D search regions anchored at the lowest and highest rib contained in $L$ (Fig. 2(c)). The initial location of the search fan is 10 mm distal from the rib starting point at the spine. The rib tangential vector at this point is used as normal vector of the fan plane. The fan opening direction withing this plane is steered by the intersection point of the previous rib with the fan plane. If only one traced rib is available yet, the fan is simply pointing upward or downward. If a neighboring rib could be found within the fan, the iterative scheme described above is applied to trace the rib. If not, the search fan is moved along the rib in 10 mm steps towards the distal end.

**Step 4: Rib Labeling.** After extraction of the centerlines, the average probability for all three non-background classes is calculated for each found rib. In the optimal case, 12 rib pairs have been found and the first and twelfth rib have an average probability along their centerlines above 0.5 for their respective class.

In this case, the intermediate ribs are labeled according to their position in the list $L$. In case that less than 12 ribs were traced, the labeling is still possible if either the first or twelfth rib can be identified. Labeling is not possible if both first and twelfth rib cannot be identified and less then 10 ribs were traced.

**Table 2.** Mean, standard deviation, 25% quartile, median and 75% quartile of the sensitivity (Sens.), precision (Prec.) and Dice score (Dice) associated to the predicted class labels *first rib*, *intermediate rib*, *twelfth rib* and the combined class *rib* across the 4 cross validation test sets.

| *first rib* | Sens. | Prec. | Dice |
|---|---|---|---|
| mean | 0.74 | 0.71 | 0.72 |
| std. | 0.09 | 0.12 | 0.10 |
| 25% qrt. | 0.70 | 0.66 | 0.69 |
| median | 0.76 | 0.73 | 0.74 |
| 75% qrt. | 0.81 | 0.78 | 0.79 |

| *twelfth rib* | Sens. | Prec. | Dice |
|---|---|---|---|
| mean | 0.69 | 0.68 | 0.61 |
| std. | 0.30 | 0.26 | 0.29 |
| 25% qrt. | 0.66 | 0.55 | 0.48 |
| median | 0.80 | 0.72 | 0.70 |
| 75% qrt. | 0.86 | 0.89 | 0.81 |

| *intermediate rib* | Sens. | Prec. | Dice |
|---|---|---|---|
| mean | 0.87 | 0.85 | 0.86 |
| std. | 0.03 | 0.05 | 0.04 |
| 25% qrt. | 0.84 | 0.83 | 0.83 |
| median | 0.87 | 0.86 | 0.87 |
| 75% qrt. | 0.90 | 0.89 | 0.89 |

| *rib* | Sens. | Prec. | Dice |
|---|---|---|---|
| mean | 0.87 | 0.85 | 0.86 |
| std. | 0.03 | 0.05 | 0.04 |
| 25% qrt. | 0.85 | 0.82 | 0.83 |
| median | 0.87 | 0.85 | 0.86 |
| 75% qrt. | 0.89 | 0.89 | 0.89 |

## 3   Results

Our pipeline was evaluated using 4-fold cross validation (CV). More precisely, the dataset was randomly shuffled and partitioned into four subsamples of sizes 28, 28, 28 and 29. We trained four different networks by using in each fold three subsamples as training data while retaining a single subsample for testing.

### 3.1   Multi-label Network

For the evaluation of a probability map $p_{ijk} = (p_{ijk,0}, p_{ijk,1}, p_{ijk,2}, p_{ijk,3})$ generated by the neural network, we assigned to each voxel $v_{ijk}$ a predicted class label $L_{ijk}^{\text{pred}}$ based on its maximal class response, i.e. $L_{ijk}^{\text{pred}} = \text{argmax}_{c=0,1,2,3} \, p_{ijk,c}$. Following the naming convention from Sect. 2.2, the labels $0, 1, 2, 3$ correspond to the classes *background*, *first rib*, *twelfth rib* and *intermediate rib*, respectively. Comparing the predicted class labels with the corresponding ground truth labels $L_{ijk}^{\text{GT}}$, yields for each class the number of true positives (TP), false positives (FP), and false negatives (FN), i.e.

$$\mathrm{TP}_C = |\{ijk \ : \ L_{ijk}^{\mathrm{GT}} = C \text{ and } L_{ijk}^{\mathrm{pred}} = C\}|,$$
$$\mathrm{FP}_C = |\{ijk \ : \ L_{ijk}^{\mathrm{GT}} \neq C \text{ and } L_{ijk}^{\mathrm{pred}} = C\}|,$$
$$\mathrm{FN}_C = |\{ijk \ : \ L_{ijk}^{\mathrm{GT}} = C \text{ and } L_{ijk}^{\mathrm{pred}} \neq C\}|,$$

where $C \in \{0, 1, 2, 3\}$ denotes the class under consideration. Henceforth, we will omit the class index $C$ in order to simplify the notation. Based on these quantities we compute for each class sensitivity, precision and Dice as follows:

$$\text{sensitivity} = \frac{\mathrm{TP}}{\mathrm{TP} + \mathrm{FN}},$$
$$\text{precision} = \frac{\mathrm{TP}}{\mathrm{TP} + \mathrm{FP}}, \tag{1}$$
$$\text{Dice} = \frac{2\mathrm{TP}}{2\mathrm{TP} + \mathrm{FP} + \mathrm{FN}}.$$

Table 2 summarizes different descriptive statistics (mean, standard deviation, median and quartiles) of the measures from (1) calculated on the test sets from the 4-fold CV. In order to analyze the overall rib detection rate irrespective of the specific rib class, we introduced an addition label *rib* which was assigned to each non-background voxel.

As can be seen from Table 2, we obtain a good performance for the overall rib detection captured, for example, by a median Dice of 0.87 for the label *intermediate rib*. Let us remark that for thin objects, such as the dilated rib centerlines, the Dice score constitutes a rather sensitive measure. The results indicate that detecting the first and twelfth rib pairs is more difficult for our network. While extraction of the first rib is more challenging due to, e.g. higher noise in the upper thorax or other bony structures in close vicinity (clavicle, shoulder blades, vertebrae), the twelfth rib can be extremely short or is even sometimes entirely missing. For further illustration, Fig. 4 shows the results on selected representative cases. Generally, the ribs are well detected without major false responses in other structures - despite all the different challenges present in the data. The color coding highlighting of the multi-label detection reveals that first and twelfth are mostly correctly detected. In few cases the network wrongly generated strong responses of the classes *first rib* or *last rib* for voxels belonging to the second or eleventh rib pair.

## 3.2 Rib Centerlines

For the evaluation of the final centerlines, both ground truth lines and automatically determined centerlines were resampled to 1.0 mm uniform point distance. A *true positive distance* of $\delta = 5.0$ mm was chosen such that, if for a ground truth point (GTP) no result point within $\delta$ was found, the GTP was counted as FN. Result points having a corresponding GTP within $\delta$ were counted as TP, all other as FP. From the TP, FP, and FN values we calculated sensitivity, precision and Dice using (1).

**Table 3.** Rib-wise evaluation of the method based on the final labeled centerline point sets. A detected rib centerline point counts only as true positive if the correct label was determined. The table shows the summary for the collected 113 cases and reports sensitivity (Sens.), precision (Prec.), point-to-line distance (Dist., in mm) and Dice score (Dice).

| Rib | Sens. | Prec. | Dist. (mm) | Dice |
|---|---|---|---|---|
| 01l | 0.924 | 0.95 | 1.34 | 0.937 |
| 01r | 0.917 | 0.95 | 1.26 | 0.933 |
| 02l | 0.978 | 0.983 | 0.83 | 0.981 |
| 02r | 0.972 | 0.970 | 0.799 | 0.971 |
| 03l | 0.991 | 0.992 | 0.721 | 0.992 |
| 03r | 0.981 | 0.980 | 0.777 | 0.981 |
| 04l | 0.994 | 0.996 | 0.681 | 0.995 |
| 04r | 0.970 | 0.983 | 0.712 | 0.977 |
| 05l | 0.995 | 0.995 | 0.695 | 0.995 |
| 05r | 0.971 | 0.975 | 0.706 | 0.973 |
| 06l | 0.995 | 0.989 | 0.682 | 0.992 |
| 06r | 0.962 | 0.963 | 0.694 | 0.963 |
| 07l | 0.991 | 0.989 | 0.680 | 0.990 |
| 07r | 0.966 | 0.957 | 0.669 | 0.961 |
| 08l | 0.991 | 0.980 | 0.666 | 0.986 |
| 08r | 0.967 | 0.961 | 0.668 | 0.964 |
| 09l | 0.993 | 0.990 | 0.685 | 0.991 |
| 09r | 0.970 | 0.966 | 0.648 | 0.968 |
| 10l | 0.991 | 0.989 | 0.676 | 0.990 |
| 10r | 0.964 | 0.961 | 0.627 | 0.963 |
| 11l | 0.985 | 0.974 | 0.711 | 0.980 |
| 11r | 0.967 | 0.960 | 0.638 | 0.964 |
| 12l | 0.956 | 0.976 | 0.873 | 0.967 |
| 12r | 0.918 | 0.947 | 0.795 | 0.933 |
| All ribs | 0.977 | 0.977 | 0.723 | 0.977 |

Tables 3 and 4 summarize our results from the 4-fold cross-validation. The point wise responses (TP, FP, FN) are averaged up over all cases. The evaluation measures are finally reported on a per rib basis, as well as for all ribs. The Euclidean distance is measured as point-to-line distance (in millimeters) between result point and ground truth line. Moreover, Table 5 contains the percentage of cases with missed labeled ribs. Here, a rib is counted as missed, if only less than half of the ground truth rib centerline could be detected. A detected rib centerline point counts only as true positive if the correct label was determined.

**Table 4.** Rib-wise evaluation of the method based on the final centerline point sets, irrespective labeling. A detected rib centerline point counts as true positive if it is close enough to a ground truth centerline, *irrespective labeling*. The table shows the summary for the collected 113 cases and reports sensitivity (Sens.), precision (Prec.), point-to-line distance (Dist., in mm) and Dice score (Dice).

| Rib | Sens. | Prec. | Dist. (mm) | Dice |
|---|---|---|---|---|
| 01l | 0.924 | 0.95 | 1.340 | 0.937 |
| 01r | 0.918 | 0.952 | 1.258 | 0.935 |
| 02l | 0.978 | 0.983 | 0.831 | 0.981 |
| 02r | 0.983 | 0.987 | 0.792 | 0.985 |
| 03l | 0.991 | 0.992 | 0.721 | 0.992 |
| 03r | 0.991 | 0.990 | 0.770 | 0.990 |
| 04l | 0.994 | 0.996 | 0.681 | 0.995 |
| 04r | 0.980 | 0.996 | 0.706 | 0.988 |
| 05l | 0.995 | 0.995 | 0.695 | 0.995 |
| 05r | 0.990 | 0.994 | 0.706 | 0.992 |
| 06l | 0.995 | 0.989 | 0.682 | 0.992 |
| 06r | 0.989 | 0.990 | 0.690 | 0.990 |
| 07l | 0.991 | 0.989 | 0.680 | 0.990 |
| 07r | 0.993 | 0.984 | 0.668 | 0.988 |
| 08l | 0.991 | 0.980 | 0.666 | 0.986 |
| 08r | 0.993 | 0.987 | 0.668 | 0.990 |
| 09l | 0.993 | 0.990 | 0.685 | 0.991 |
| 09r | 0.996 | 0.992 | 0.651 | 0.994 |
| 10l | 0.991 | 0.990 | 0.677 | 0.991 |
| 10r | 0.989 | 0.985 | 0.630 | 0.987 |
| 11l | 0.985 | 0.975 | 0.713 | 0.981 |
| 11r | 0.988 | 0.980 | 0.645 | 0.984 |
| 12l | 0.956 | 0.976 | 0.873 | 0.967 |
| 12r | 0.932 | 0.961 | 0.798 | 0.947 |
| All ribs | 0.986 | 0.987 | 0.722 | 0.987 |

**Table 5.** Percentage of cases with missed labeled ribs. A rib counts as missed, if less than half of the ground truth rib centerline could be detected. A detected rib centerline point counts only as true positive if the correct label was determined.

| No. missed ribs | Case percentage |
|---|---|
| 0 | 85.8% |
| 1 | 5.3% |
| 2 | 6.2% |
| $\geq 3$ | 2.6% |

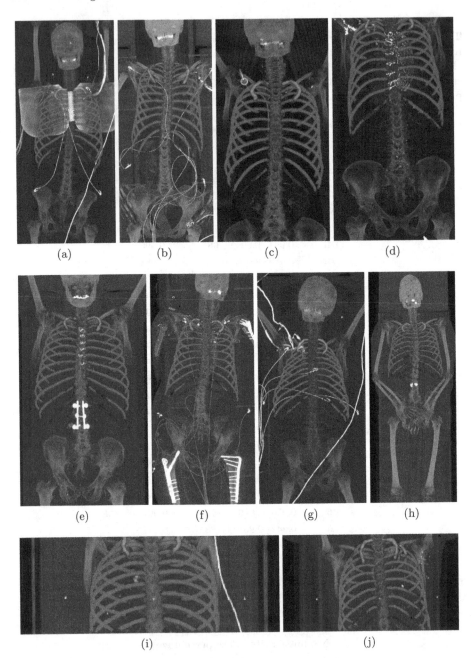

**Fig. 4.** Maximum intensity projections of selected computed tomography volumes overlaid with the multi-label output of the neural network (green: first rib; red: intermediate rib; blue: twelfth rib). The selected case above display common difficulties which are inherent in the data set, such as (a) pads or (b) cables, internal devices such as (c) pacemakers, (d) stents, (e) spinal implants, (f) femoral/humeral implants, (g) injected contrast agents, (h) patient shape variations such as scoliosis, and limited field of views, i.e. (i) partly missing first rib or (j) partly missing twelfth rib. (Color figure online)

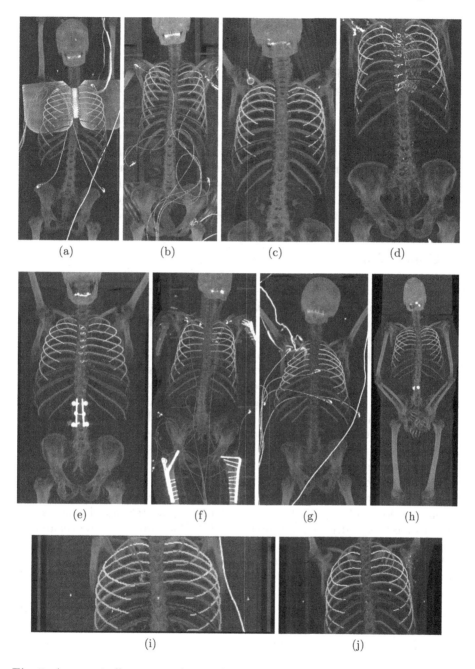

**Fig. 5.** Automatically generated centerline splines associated with the fully convolutional neural network outputs displayed in Fig. 4. The selected case above display common difficulties which are inherent in the data set, such as (a) pads or (b) cables, internal devices such as (c) pacemakers, (d) stents, (e) spinal implants and (f) femural/humeral implants, (g) injected contrast agents, (h) patient shape variations such as scoliosis, limited field of views, i.e. (i) partly missing first rib or (j) twelfth rib.

With an average Euclidean distance error of 0.723 mm, we obtained an overall result that is generally better compared to what is reported in the state of the art. Although, it needs to be kept in mind that results are unfortunately not directly comparable as both the data sets as well the evaluation metrics significantly differ across prior work. Similarly to the results obtained on the probability maps, distance errors are significantly higher for first and twelfth rib compared to the rest of the rib cage. As discussed, this is caused by the intrinsic challenges of these ribs, but certainly also an affect of error propagation in that sense that the quality of the probability maps also impacts centerline extraction. Interestingly, the right ribs are generally slightly worse compared to the left ribs, probably due to a slightly unbalanced data set with more challenges on the right side. Figure 5 shows the centerlines which were automatically generated using our walker algorithm from the corresponding network outputs displayed in Fig. 4.

## 4   Conclusion

We presented a fully automated two-stage approach for rib centerline extraction and labeling from CT images. First, multi-label probability maps (containing the classes first rib, twelfth rib, intermediate ribs, background) are calculated using a FCNN and then centerlines are extracted from this multi-label information using a tracing algorithm. For assessment, we performed a 4-fold cross validation on a set of 113 cases which includes several cases displaying typical clinical challenges. Comparing the automated extraction results to our manual ground truth annotations, we were able to achieve an Euclidean point-to-line distance error of 0.723 mm. The 4-class label detection was crucial to simplify rib labeling by taking the network responses associated to the classes *first rib* and *twelfth rib* into account. In contrast to other approaches, no strong anatomical prior knowledge, e.g. in the form of geometrical models, was explicitly encoded into our pipeline to deal with pathological deviations.

Future work will focus on improving the performance of the neural network by using motion field and registration based data augmentation techniques and a more advanced data-driven image preprocessing which aims at better separating foreground and background voxels.

We would like to mention that the approach outlined above was already extended by training the FCNN to segment a dilated spinal column centerline in addition to the dilated rib centerlines. This additional information is utilized by the walker algorithm in order to generate a spinal column centerline which is subsequently used to improve the performance of the rib tracing, for example by detecting wrongly labeled rib pairs.

# References

1. Tobon-Gomez, C., et al.: Unfolded cylindrical projection for rib fracture diagnosis. In: Glocker, B., Yao, J., Vrtovec, T., Frangi, A., Zheng, G. (eds.) MSKI 2017. LNCS, vol. 10734, pp. 36–47. Springer, Cham (2018). https://doi.org/10.1007/978-3-319-74113-0_4

2. Wu, D., et al.: A learning based deformable template matching method for automatic rib centerline extraction and labeling in CT images. In: Proceedings of 2012 IEEE Conference on Computer Vision and Pattern Recognition, CVPR 2012, pp. 980–987. IEEE (2012). https://doi.org/10.1109/CVPR.2012.6247774

3. Shen, H., Liang, L., Shao, M., Qing, S.: Tracing based segmentation for the labeling of individual rib structures in chest CT volume data. In: Barillot, C., Haynor, D.R., Hellier, P. (eds.) MICCAI 2004. LNCS, vol. 3217, pp. 967–974. Springer, Heidelberg (2004). https://doi.org/10.1007/978-3-540-30136-3_117

4. Lee, J., Reeves, A.: Segmentation of individual ribs from low-dose chest CT. In: Karssemeijer, N., Summers, R. (eds.) Proceedings of SPIE Medical Imaging 2010: Computer Aided Diagnosis, vol. 7624, p. 76243J. SPIE (2010). https://doi.org/10.1117/12.844565

5. Staal, J., van Ginneken, B., Viergever, M.: Automatic ribsegmentation and labeling in computed tomography scans using ageneral framework for detection, recognition and segmentation ofobjects in volumetric data. Med. Image Anal. 11(1), 35–46 (2006). https://doi.org/10.1016/j.media.2006.10.001

6. Klinder, T., Lorenz, C., von Berg, J., Dries, S.P.M., Bülow, T., Ostermann, J.: Automated model-based rib cage segmentation and labeling in CT images. In: Ayache, N., Ourselin, S., Maeder, A. (eds.) MICCAI 2007. LNCS, vol. 4792, pp. 195–202. Springer, Heidelberg (2007). https://doi.org/10.1007/978-3-540-75759-7_24

7. Brosch, T., Saalbach, A.: Foveal fully convolutional nets for multi-organ segmentation. In: Angelini, E., Landman, B. (eds.) Proceedings of SPIE Medical Imaging 2018: Image Processing, vol. 10574, p. 105740U. SPIE (2018). https://doi.org/10.1117/12.2293528

8. Zeiler, M.: ADADELTA: an adaptive learning rate method. arXiv:1212.5701 (2012)

# Automatic Detection of Wrist Fractures From Posteroanterior and Lateral Radiographs: A Deep Learning-Based Approach

Raja Ebsim[1](✉), Jawad Naqvi[2], and Timothy F. Cootes[1]

[1] Centre for Imaging Sciences, The University of Manchester, Manchester, UK
raja.ebsim@manchester.ac.uk
[2] Health Education North West School of Radiology, Manchester, UK

**Abstract.** We present a system that uses convolutional neural networks (CNNs) to detect wrist fractures (distal radius fractures) in posterioanterior and lateral radiographs. The proposed system uses random forest regression voting constrained local model to automatically segment the radius. The resulting automatic annotation is used to register the object across the dataset and crop patches. A CNN is trained on the registered patches for each view separately. Our automatic system outperformed existing systems with a performance of 96% (area under receiver operating characteristic curve) on cross-validation experiments on a dataset of 1010 patients, half of them with fractures.

**Keywords:** Medical image analysis with deep learning
X-ray fracture detection · Wrist fracture detection
Computer-aided diagnosis

## 1 Introduction

Wrist fractures are the commonest type of fractures seen in emergency departments (EDs), They are estimated to be 18% of the fractures seen in adults [1,2] and of 25% of fractures seen in children [2]. They are usually identified in EDs by doctors examining lateral (LAT) and posterioanterior (PA) radiographs. Yet wrist fractures are one of the most commonly-missed in ED-examined radiographs [3,4]. Systems that can identify suspicious wrist areas and notify ED staff could reduce the number of misdiagnoses.

In this paper we describe a fully-automated system for detecting radius fractures in PA and LAT radiographs. For each view, a global search [5] is performed for finding the approximate position of the radius. The detailed outline of the bone is then located using a random forest regression voting constrained local model (RFCLM) [6]. Convolutional neural networks (CNNs) are trained on cropped patches containing the region of interest on the task of detecting fractures. The decisions from both views are averaged for better performance. This

© Springer Nature Switzerland AG 2019
T. Vrtovec et al. (Eds.): MSKI 2018, LNCS 11404, pp. 114–125, 2019.
https://doi.org/10.1007/978-3-030-11166-3_10

paper is the first to show an automatic system for identifying fractures from PA and LAT view radiographs of the wrist by using convolutional neural networks, outperforming previously-published works.

## 2 Previous Work

Early work on fracture detection used non-visual techniques: analysing mechanical vibration [7], analysing acoustic waves travelling along the bone [8], or by measuring electrical conductivity [9]. The first published work on detecting fractures in radiographs was that in [10] where an algorithm is developed to measure the femur neckshaft angle and use it to determine whether the femur is fractured. There is a body of literature on radiographic fracture detection on a variety of anatomical regions, including arm fractures [11], femur fractures [10, 12–15], and vertebral endplates [16]. Cao et al. [17] worked on fractures in a range of different anatomical regions using stacked random forests to fuse different feature representations (Schmid texture feature, Gabor texture feature, and forward contextual-intensity). They achieved a sensitivity of 81% and precision of 25%. Work on wrist fracture detection from radiographs is still limited. The earliest works [13, 14] used active shape models and active appearance models [18] to locate the approximate contour of the radius and trained support vector machine (SVM) on extracted texture features (Gabor, Markov random field, and gradient intensity). They worked on a small dataset with only 23 fractured examples in their test set and achieved encouraging performance. In previous work [19, 20] we used RFCLMs [21] to segment the radius in PA and LAT views and trained random forest (RF) classifiers on statistical shape parameters and eigen-mode texture features [18]. The fully automated system achieved a performance of 91.4% (area under receiver operating characteristic curve, AUC) on a dataset of 787 radiographs (378 of which were fractured) in cross-validation experiments and was the first to combine the both views. Instead of hand-crafting features Kim et al. [22] re-trained the top layer (i.e. classifier) of inception v3 network [23] to detect fractures in wrist LAT views from features previously-learned from non-radiological images (ImageNet [24]). This was the first work to use deep learning in the task of detecting wrist fractures. The system was tested on 100 images (half of which fractured) and reported an AUC of 95.4%. However, they excluded images where lateral projection was inconclusive for the presence or absence of fracture which would bias the results favourably but contradict the goal of developing such systems (i.e. helping clinicians with difficult usually-missed fractures). Olczak et al. [25] re-trained five common deep networks from Caffe library [26] on dataset of 256,000 wrist, hand, and ankle radiographs, of which 56% of the images contained fractures. The dataset was divided into (70% training, 20% validation, and 10% testing) and used to train the networks for the tasks of detecting fractures, determining which exam view, body part, and laterality (left or right). Labels were extracted by automatically mining reports and DICOMs. The images were rescaled to $256 \times 256$ and then cropped into a subsection of the original image with the network's input size.

The pre-processing causes image distortion but they justified that as the nature of tasks does not need non-distorted images. The networks were pre-trained on the ImageNet dataset [24] and then their top layers (i.e. classifier) were replaced with fully connected layers suitable for each task. The best performing network (VGG 16 [27]) achieved a fracture detection accuracy of 83% without reporting false positive rate. The model deals with various views independently but it does not combine them for a decision. Another related work [28] used a very deep CNN-based model (169 trainable layers) for abnormality detection from raw radiographs. Images are labelled as normal or abnormal, where abnormal does not always mean "fractured" - it sometimes means there is metalwork present. Their dataset contains metal hardware in both categories (normal and abnormal) and also contains different age groups. This makes the definition of abnormality is rather unclear as what is considered abnormal for a certain group can be seen as normal for another age group and vice versa.

## 3   Background

### 3.1   Shape Modeling and Matching

Statistical shape models (SSMs) [18] are widely used for studying the contours of bones. Shape is the quality left after all differences due to location, orientation, and scale are omitted in a population of same-class objects. SSMs assume that each shape instance is a deformed version of the mean shape describing the object class. The training data is used to identify the mean shape and its possible deformations. The contour of an object is described by a set of model points $(x_i, y_i)$ packed in a $2n$-D vector $\mathbf{x} = (x_1, \ldots, x_n, y_1, \ldots, y_n)^T$. An SSM is a linear model of shape variations of the object across the training dataset built by applying principal component analysis (PCA) to aligned shapes and fitting a Gaussian distribution in the reduced space. A shape instance $\mathbf{x}$ is represented as:

$$\mathbf{x} \approx T_\theta(\bar{\mathbf{x}} + \mathbf{Pb} : \theta), \tag{1}$$

where $\bar{\mathbf{x}}$ is the mean shape, $\mathbf{P}$ is the set of the orthogonal eigenvectors corresponding to the $t$ highest eigenvalues of the covariance matrix of the training data, $\mathbf{b}$ is the vector of shape parameters and $T(. : \theta)$ applies a similarity transformation with parameters $\theta$ between the common reference frame and the image frame. The number of the used eigenvectors $t$ is chosen to represent most of the total variation (i.e. 95–98%).

One of the most effective algorithms for locating the outline of bones in radiographs is RFCLM [6]. This uses a collection of RFs to predict the most likely location of each point based on nearby image patches. A shape model is then used to constrain the points and encode the result.

### 3.2   Convolutional Neural Network

CNNs are a class of deep feed-forward artificial neural networks for processing data that has a known grid-like topology. They emerged from the study of the brain's visual cortex and benefited from the recent increase in the computational power and the amount of available training data.

A typical CNN (Fig. 1) stacks few convolutional layers, then followed by a subsampling layer (*Pooling layer*), then another few convolutional layers, then another pooling layer, and so on. At the top of the stack fully-connected layers are added outputing a prediction (e.g. estimated class probabilities). This layer-wise fashion allows CNNs to combine low-level features to form higher-level features (Fig. 2), learning features and eliminating the need for hand crafted feature extractors. In addition, the learned features are translation invariant, incorporating the two-dimensional (2D) spatial structure of images which contributed to CNNs achieving state-of-the-art results in image-related tasks.

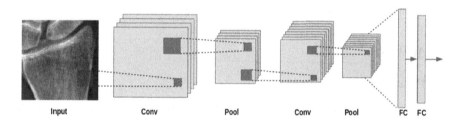

**Fig. 1.** A convolutional neural network-based classifier applied to a single-channel input image. Every convolutional layer (Conv) transforms its input to a three-dimensional output volume of neuron activations. The pooling layer (Pool) downsamples the volume spatially, independently in each feature map of its input volume. At the end fully-connected layers (FC) output a prediction.

A convolutional layer has $k$ filters (or kernels) of size $r \times r \times c$ (receptive field size) where $r$ is smaller than the input width/height, and $c$ is the same as the input depth. Every filter convolves with the input volume in sliding-window fashion to produce feature maps (Fig. 2). Each convolution operation is followed by a nonlinear activation, typically a rectified linear unit (ReLU) which sets any negative values to zero. A feature map can be subsampled by taking the mean or maximum value over $p \times p$ contiguous regions to produce translation invariant features (Pooling). The value of $p$ usually ranges between 2–5 depending on how large the input is. This reduction in spatial size leads to fewer parameters, less computation, and controls overfitting.

The local connections, tied weights, and pooling result in CNNs have fewer trainable parameters than fully connected networks with the same number of hidden units. The parameters are learned by back propagation with gradient-based optimization to reduce a cost function.

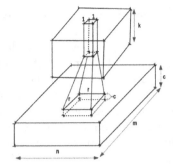

**Fig. 2.** In the convolutional neural network, $k$ neurons receive input from only a restricted subarea (receptive field) of the previous layer output. Convolving the filters with the whole input volume produces $k$ feature maps.

## 4   Methods

### 4.1   Patch Preparation

Because most parts of a radiograph are either background or irrelevant to the task, we chose to train CNNs on cropped patches rather than raw images. The steps of the automated system are shown in Fig. 3. Following our previous work [20] we used a global search with a random forest regression voting (RFRV) technique to find the approximate radius location (red dots in Fig. 3) followed by a local search performed by a sequence of RFCLM models with an increasing resolution to find its contour. The automatic point annotation gives information on the position, orientation and scale of the distal radius accurately. This is used to transfer the bone to a standardized coordinate frame before cropping a patch of size ($n_i \times n_i$ pixels) containing the bone. We used the resulting patches to train and test a CNN. This process is completely automatic. Figure 4 shows examples of radiographs and extracted patches.

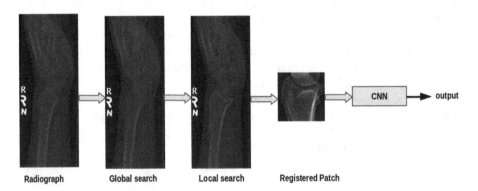

Radiograph      Global search      Local search      Registered Patch

**Fig. 3.** Fully automated system for detecting wrist fractures. (Color figure online)

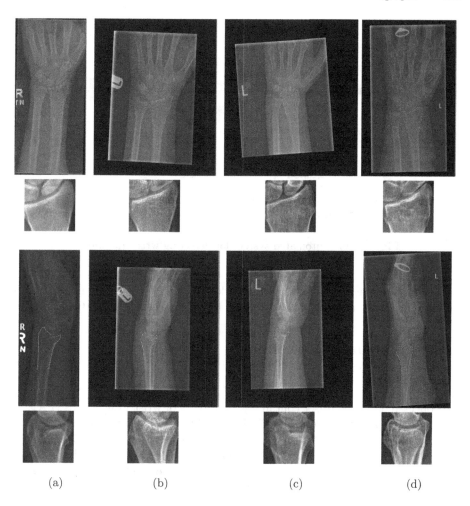

**Fig. 4.** Example of pairs of radiographs for four subjects with (a) a normal radius, (b)–(d) fracture radiuses. The first and third rows show the posterioanterior and lateral views respectively. The corresponding cropped patches appear below each view.

## 4.2   Network Architecture

We trained a CNN for each view. The two CNNs were classical stacks of CP layers (CP refers to one ReLU-activated convolutional layer followed by a pooling layer) with two consecutive fully-connected (FC) layers. No padding was used. Weights were initialised with the Xavier uniform kernel initializer [29] and biases initialised to zeros. The loss function was binary cross entropy optimised with Adam [30] (default parameter values used). An input patch size of $121 \times 121$, and of $151 \times 151$ were used for PA, and LAT networks respectively. Architecture details are summarised in Table 1. In our experiments we gradually increased the

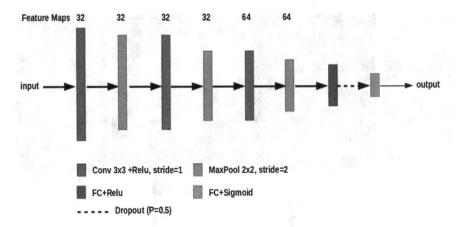

**Fig. 5.** Fully automated system for detecting wrist fractures.

number of CP layers and chose the network with the best performance. Figure 5 shows an example network with three CP layers followed by two FC layers.

## 5    Experiments and Results

### 5.1    Data

We collected a wrist dataset containing 1010 pairs of wrist radiographs (PA and LAT) for 1010 adult patients, 505 of whom had fractures (Fig. 4). Images for 787 patients, 378 of whom had fractures, were gathered from two local EDs while the rest were gathered from the MURA dataset [28] with fractures as abnormality. Fractured examples do not contain any plaster casts or metalware to make sure the network learns features for detecting fracture not hardware.

### 5.2    Fracture Detection

We carried out 5-fold cross validation experiments. During each fold 802 radio-graphs were used as training set, 102 as validation set, and 102 as testing set. The validation and testing sets were then swapped so that all the data were tested exactly once. Every time a network was trained from scratch for 20 epochs with batch size = 32 and the model with the lowest validation loss was selected. Training data was randomly shuffled at the start of each epoch to produce different batches each time. We found the architectures with three CP layers, and with four CP layers performed the best for the LAT view, and PA view respectively. Having trained the two CNNs, one for each view, their outputs are combined by averaging (Fig. 6). Figure 7 shows the average performance and learning curves. We achieved an average performance of AUC = 95% for PA view, 93% for LAT view, and 96% from both views combined.

**Table 1.** The overall architecture detailed with maps' sizes corresponding to an input wrist patch of size $121 \times 121$. Same architecture also used with $151 \times 151$. In our experiments we gradually increased the number of CP layers and chose the network with the best performance.

| Layer | Type | Maps | Size | Kernel size | Stride | Activation |
|---|---|---|---|---|---|---|
| In | Input | 1 | $121 \times 121$ | - | - | - |
| CP1 | Convolution | 32 | $119 \times 119$ | $3 \times 3$ | 1 | Relu |
| | Max pooling 2D | 32 | $59 \times 59$ | $2 \times 2$ | 2 | - |
| CP2 | Convolution | 32 | $57 \times 57$ | $3 \times 3$ | 1 | Relu |
| | Max pooling 2D | 32 | $28 \times 28$ | $2 \times 2$ | 2 | - |
| CP3 | Convolution | 64 | $26 \times 26$ | $3 \times 3$ | 1 | Relu |
| | Max pooling 2D | 64 | $13 \times 13$ | $2 \times 2$ | 2 | - |
| CP4 | Convolution | 64 | $11 \times 11$ | $3 \times 3$ | 1 | Relu |
| | Max pooling 2D | 64 | $5 \times 5$ | $2 \times 2$ | 2 | - |
| CP5 | Convolution | 64 | $3 \times 3$ | $3 \times 3$ | 1 | Relu |
| | Max pooling 2D | 64 | $1 \times 1$ | $2 \times 2$ | 2 | - |
| FC1 | Fully connected | - | 64 | - | - | Relu |
| D | Dropout (rate $= 0.5$) | - | - | - | - | - |
| FC2 | Fully connected | - | 1 | - | - | Sigmoid |

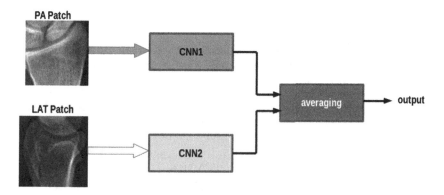

**Fig. 6.** During testing the outputs for both views are combined by averaging.

Kim et al. [22] used features originally learned to classify non-radiological images [24] and used them to detect fractures in LAT views and reported an AUC of 95.4%. Unlike their work we have not excluded images where lateral projection was inconclusive for the presence or absence of fracture which would bias the results favourably. In our case, we performed 5-fold cross-validation and reported an overall AUC of 96%. For the sake of comparison with our previous RF-based technique in [20] we repeated all experiments in [20] on the current dataset with the same fold divisions and found an AUC of 92% from two views

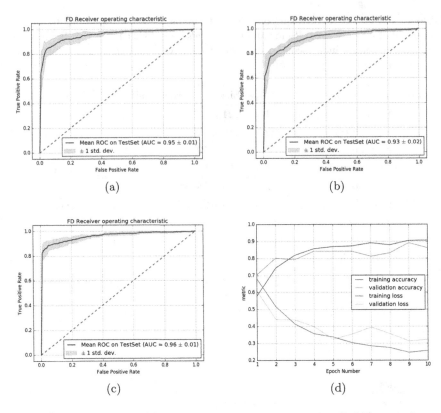

**Fig. 7.** Fracture detection. (a) Receiver operating characteristic (ROC) curve for posterioanterior view. (b) ROC curve for lateral view. (c) ROC curve for both views combined. (d) Example of learning curves for a model.

**Table 2.** Comparison between convolutional neural network (CNN)-based and random forest (RF)-based techniques on the same dataset in terms of area under the curve ± standard deviation (PA - posteroanterior, LAT - lateral).

| Method | PA view | LAT view | Both views |
|---|---|---|---|
| CNNs | $0.95 \pm 0.01$ | $0.93 \pm 0.02$ | $0.96 \pm 0.01$ |
| RFs on shape and texture params [20] | $0.89 \pm 0.02$ | $0.91 \pm 0.02$ | $0.92 \pm 0.02$ |

combined, 89% and 91% for PA view, and LAT view respectively (Table 2 and Fig. 8). The CNN-based technique clearly outperforms the RF-based one.

## 5.3   Conclusions

We presented a system for automatic wrist fracture detection from plain PA and LAT X-rays. The CNN is trained from scratch on radiographic patches cropped around the joint after automatic segmentation and registration. This directed

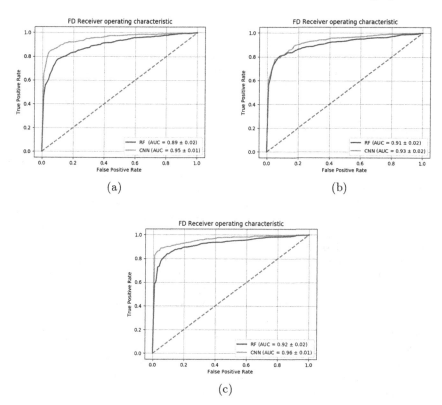

**Fig. 8.** Comparison between receiver operating characteristics curves for the proposed convolutional neural network-based technique and the relevant random forest-based work in [20] on: (a) posteroanterior view, (b) lateral view, and (c) both views combined for the same dataset in terms of area under the curve ± standard deviation.

preprocessing ensures meaningful learning from only the targeted region in scale which in turn reduces the noise a CNN is exposed to compared to when trained on full images containing parts that are not relevant to the task. Radiographs, unlike photos, have predictable contents that allow model-based techniques to work well and therefore they can provide CNNs with an input that dispense with the need to: (1) perform any data augmentation and (2) unnecessarily complicate the deep architecture and its learning process. Our work was the first to train CNNs from scratch on the task of detecting wrist fractures and to combine the two views for a decision. The experiments showed that combining the results from both views leads to an improvement in overall classification performance, with an AUC of 96% compared to 95% for PA view and 93% for LAT view.

**Acknowledgements.** The research leading to these results has received funding from Libyan Ministry of Higher Education and Research. The authors would like to thank Dr Jonathan Harris, Dr Matthew Davenport, and Dr Martin Smith for their help setting up the project.

# References

1. Court-Brown, C., Caesar, B.: Epidemiology of adult fractures: a review. Injury **37**(8), 691–697 (2006). https://doi.org/10.1016/j.injury.2006.04.130
2. Goldfarb, C., Yin, Y., Gilula, L., Fisher, A., Boyer, M.: Wrist fractures: what the clinician wants to know. Radiology **219**(1), 11–28 (2001). https://doi.org/10.1148/radiology.219.1.r01ap1311
3. Guly, H.: Injuries initially misdiagnosed as sprained wrist (beware the sprained wrist). Emerg. Med. J. **19**(1), 41–42 (2002). https://doi.org/10.1136/emj.19.1.41
4. Petinaux, B., Bhat, R., Boniface, K., Aristizabal, J.: Accuracy of radiographic readings in the emergency department. Am. J. Emerg. Med. **29**(1), 18–25 (2011). https://doi.org/10.1016/j.ajem.2009.07.011
5. Lindner, C., Thiagarajah, S., Wilkinson, J., Wallis, G., Cootes, T., The arcOGEN Consortium: Fully automatic segmentation of the proximal femur using random forest regression voting. IEEE Trans. Med. Imaging **32**(8), 1462–1472 (2013). https://doi.org/10.1109/TMI.2013.2258030
6. Cootes, T.F., Ionita, M.C., Lindner, C., Sauer, P.: Robust and accurate shape model fitting using random forest regression voting. In: Fitzgibbon, A., Lazebnik, S., Perona, P., Sato, Y., Schmid, C. (eds.) ECCV 2012. LNCS, vol. 7578, pp. 278–291. Springer, Heidelberg (2012). https://doi.org/10.1007/978-3-642-33786-4_21
7. Kaufman, J., et al.: A neural network approach for bone fracture healing assessment. IEEE Eng. Med. Biol. Mag. **9**(3), 23–30 (1990). https://doi.org/10.1109/51.59209
8. Ryder, D., King, S., Oliff, C., Davies, E.: A possible method of monitoring bone fracture and bone characteristics using a noninvasive acoustic technique. In: Proceedings of International Conference on Acoustic Sensing and Imaging, pp. 159–163. IEEE (1993)
9. Singh, V., Chauhan, S.: Early detection of fracture healing of a long bone for better mass health care. In: Proceedings of 20th International Conference of the Engineering in Medicine and Biology Society – EMBC 1998, vol. 6, pp. 2911–2912. IEEE (1998). https://doi.org/10.1109/IEMBS.1998.746096
10. Tian, T.P., Chen, Y., Leow, W.K., Hsu, W., Howe, T.S., Png, M.A.: Computing neck-shaft angle of femur for X-ray fracture detection. In: Petkov, N., Westenberg, M.A. (eds.) CAIP 2003. LNCS, vol. 2756, pp. 82–89. Springer, Heidelberg (2003). https://doi.org/10.1007/978-3-540-45179-2_11
11. Jia, Y., Jiang, Y.: Active contour model with shape constraints for bone fracture detection. In: Proceedings of 3rd International Conference on Computer Graphics, Imaging and Visualisation – CGIV 2006, pp. 90–95. IEEE (2006). https://doi.org/10.1109/CGIV.2006.16
12. Yap, D.H., Chen, Y., Leow, W., Howe, T., Png, M.: Detecting femur fractures by texture analysis of trabeculae. In: Proceedings of 17th International Conference on Pattern Recognition – ICPR 2004, vol. 3, pp. 730–733. IEEE (2004). https://doi.org/10.1109/ICPR.2004.1334632
13. Lim, S., Xing, Y., Chen, Y., Leow, W., Howe, T., Png, M.: Detection of femur and radius fractures in X-ray images. In: Proceedings of 2nd International Conference on Advances in Medical Signal and Information Processing, pp. 249–256 (2004)
14. Lum, V., Leow, W., Chen, Y., Howe, T., Png, M.: Combining classifiers for bone fracture detection in X-ray images. In: Proceedings of International Conference on Image Processing – ICIP 2005, p. I-1149. IEEE (2005). https://doi.org/10.1109/ICIP.2005.1529959

15. Bayram, F., Çakiroğlu, M.: DIFFRACT: DIaphyseal Femur FRActure Classifier SysTem. Biocybern. Biomed. Eng. **36**(1), 157–171 (2016). https://doi.org/10.1016/j.bbe.2015.10.003

16. Roberts, M., Oh, T., Pacheco, E., Mohankumar, R., Cootes, T., Adams, J.: Semi-automatic determination of detailed vertebral shape from lumbar radiographs using active appearance models. Osteoporos. Int. **23**(2), 655–664 (2012). https://doi.org/10.1007/s00198-011-1604-3

17. Cao, Y., Wang, H., Moradi, M., Prasanna, P., Syeda-Mahmood, T.: Fracture detection in X-ray images through stacked random forests feature fusion. In: Proceedings of 12th International Symposium on Biomedical Imaging – ISBI 2015, pp. 801–805. IEEE (2015). https://doi.org/10.1109/ISBI.2015.7163993

18. Cootes, T., Edwards, G., Taylor, C.: Active appearance models. IEEE Trans. Pattern Anal. Mach. Intell. **23**(6), 681–685 (2001). https://doi.org/10.1109/34.927467

19. Ebsim, R., Naqvi, J., Cootes, T.: Detection of wrist fractures in X-ray images. In: Shekhar, R., et al. (eds.) CLIP 2016. LNCS, vol. 9958, pp. 1–8. Springer, Cham (2016). https://doi.org/10.1007/978-3-319-46472-5_1

20. Ebsim, R., Naqvi, J., Cootes, T.: Fully automatic detection of distal radius fractures from posteroanterior and lateral radiographs. In: Cardoso, M.J., et al. (eds.) CARE/CLIP - 2017. LNCS, vol. 10550, pp. 91–98. Springer, Cham (2017). https://doi.org/10.1007/978-3-319-67543-5_8

21. Lindner, C., Bromiley, P., Ionita, M., Cootes, T.: Robust and accurate shape model matching using random forest regression-voting. IEEE Trans. Pattern Anal. Mach. Intell. **37**(9), 1862–1874 (2015). https://doi.org/10.1109/TPAMI.2014.2382106

22. Kim, D., MacKinnon, T.: Artificial intelligence in fracture detection: transfer learning from deep convolutional neural networks. Clin. Radiol. **73**(5), 439–445 (2018). https://doi.org/10.1016/j.crad.2017.11.015

23. Szegedy, C., Vanhoucke, V., Ioffe, S., Shlens, J., Wojna, Z.: Rethinking the inception architecture for computer vision. In: Proceedings of 29th IEEE Conference on Computer Vision and Pattern Recognition – CVPR 2016, pp. 2818–2826. IEEE (2016). https://doi.org/10.1109/CVPR.2016.308

24. Russakovsky, O., et al.: ImageNet large scale visual recognition challenge. Int. J. Comput. Vis. **115**(3), 211–252 (2015). https://doi.org/10.1007/s11263-015-0816-y

25. Olczak, J., et al.: Artificial intelligence for analyzing orthopedic trauma radiographs: deep learning algorithms—are they on par with humans for diagnosing fractures? Acta Orthop. **88**(6), 581–586 (2017). https://doi.org/10.1080/17453674.2017.1344459

26. Jia, Y., et al.: Caffe: convolutional architecture for fast feature embedding. In: Proceedings of 22nd International Conference on Multimedia – MM 2014, pp. 675–678. ACM (2014). https://doi.org/10.1145/2647868.2654889

27. Zhong, S., Li, K., Feng, R.: Deep convolutional hamming ranking network for large scale image retrieval. In: Proceedings of 11th World Congress on Intelligent Control and Automation – WCICA 2014, pp. 1018–1023. IEEE (2014). https://doi.org/10.1109/WCICA.2014.7052856

28. Rajpurkar, P., et al.: MURA large dataset for abnormality detection in musculoskeletal radiographs. arXiv:1712.06957v1 (2017)

29. Glorot, X., Bengio, Y.: Understanding the difficulty of training deep feedforward neural networks. In: Teh, Y., Titterington, M. (eds.) Proceedings of 13th International Conference on Artificial Intelligence and Statistics – AISTATS 2010, PMLR, vol. 9, pp. 249–256. PMLR (2010)

30. Kingma, D., Ba, J.: Adam: a method for stochastic optimization. arXiv:1412.6980 (2014)

# Bone Reconstruction and Depth Control During Laser Ablation

Uri Nahum$^{(\boxtimes)}$, Azhar Zam, and Philippe C. Cattin

Department of Biomedical Engineering, University of Basel, Basel, Switzerland
uri.nahum@unibas.ch

**Abstract.** Cutting bones using laser light has been studied by several groups over the last decades. Yet, the risk of cutting nerves or soft tissues behind the bone is still an untackled problem. When performing tissue ablation such as bone, an acoustic signal is emitted. This paper presents a numerical framework that takes advantage of this acoustic signal to reconstruct not only the structure of the bone but also estimates the current cut position and depth. We employ an inverse problems approach to estimate the bone structure followed by an optimal control step to localize the position and depth of the signal source, i.e. the position of the cut. Besides the methodological description we also present numerical simulations in two dimensions with realistic mixed soft- and hard-tissue objects.

**Keywords:** Inverse problems · Optimal control · Laser ablation
Depth control

## 1 Introduction

Since its invention in the 1950's, researchers have dreamed of using lasers for surgical procedures: the cuts are extremely precise and the healing process is shorter with respect to sawing. Whereas soft-tissue laser applications are quite common in daily surgical routine, the introduction of lasers in cutting hard tissue has not yet happened. The main reason being that bones often carbonized during the ablation process impairing healing. Another reason is the difficulty of controlling the depth of the cut to avoid any damage to the tissue on the posterior side of the bone once cut through. In craniotomy, for example, the system has to ensure that no damage will be caused to the dura and brain when cutting through the skull bone. This is, however, an inherently difficult challenge and people have been trying to solve it with optical coherence tomography (OCT) such as in [1]. The problem with OCT is - besides its cost - that the laser only sees a couple of micrometers into the bone which is not enough when with each laser shot more than one hundred micrometers are removed.

In contrast to the more common OCT depth control solutions we propose to formulate the ablation progression in an inverse problem framework by taking advantage of the acoustic wave produced during the ablation process [2]. Such

© Springer Nature Switzerland AG 2019
T. Vrtovec et al. (Eds.): MSKI 2018, LNCS 11404, pp. 126–135, 2019.
https://doi.org/10.1007/978-3-030-11166-3_11

inverse scattering problems appear in a wide area of research, for example, radar technology, geophysical exploration and medical imaging.

In general, inverse medium problems are solved by the following strategy: a known acoustic source produces a wave which travels through the medium. The wave collects information about the medium by propagating through its layers and features or by reflecting from them. The wave and its reflections are then measured at sensors outside the medium. After collecting the data, the measurements are compared with a simulation of the wave propagating through an estimated medium, which is chosen as an initial guess. The misfit between the simulated data and the true measurements is minimized to reveal the properties and structure of the medium [3].

In the last two decades many applications, optimization methods [4–6], algorithms [7] and special bases [8,9] have been applied to the inverse medium problem. In this paper, we use the acoustic wave, produced by the laser beam when cutting the bone and apply some of the knowledge cited above to get information about the bone structure and the current depth of the cut.

## 2   Method

The propagation of acoustic waves through a medium can be described by the acoustic wave equation:

$$y_{tt}(x,t) - \nabla \cdot (u(x)\nabla y(x,t)) = f(x,t), \tag{1}$$

where $u(x) > 0$ represents the squared medium wave velocity in the different tissues and hence, is given by the bone structure. The source function $f(x,t)$ is emitted by cutting the bone with a laser beam and $y(x,t)$ the pressure variation, i.e. the wave field produced by the cut process. Hence, for a given bone structure and an acoustic source, we get a solution $y(x,t)$ which represents the wave at location $x$ and time $t$ and $y_{tt}$ denotes its second time derivative.

### 2.1   Inverse Medium Problem

Now, we assume that the bone structure $u(x)$ is unknown and we would like to reconstruct it using the acoustic wave produced by the cutting process. Therefore, we position sensors close to the source of the laser beam and denote by $y^{obs}$ the measurements at their position. We seek a reconstruction of the unknown squared wave velocity $u$ of the bone structure, such that the solution $y$ of (1) with $f$ coincides with the measurements $y^{obs}$. We follow [3,4,8] to solve the inverse medium problem and formulate it as a partial differential equation (PDE)-constrained optimization problem:

$$\text{minimize } \mathcal{F}(u,y) = \frac{1}{2}\left\| Py - y^{obs} \right\|_{L^2}^2, \tag{2}$$

such that $y(u)$ satisfies (1) for a source $f$, and $P$ is the projection at the sensor positions.

The amount of data in inverse medium problems tends to be large, especially when data is available for all time. By using the Fourier transform of the time variable, the source and the wave field can be represented by a sum of time harmonic waves. This allows us to separate time and space dimensions and write $f$ and $y$ as:

$$y(x,t) = \hat{y}(x)e^{-i\omega t} \qquad \text{and} \qquad f(x,t) = \hat{f}(x)e^{-i\omega t}, \tag{3}$$

where $\omega > 0$ denotes the time frequency. Replacing (3) in (1) leads to the Helmholtz equation (for the sake of simplicity, we now drop the hat notation from the Fourier transform):

$$-\omega^2 y(x) - \nabla \cdot (u(x)\nabla y(x)) = f(x). \tag{4}$$

In numerical computations, the infinite exterior must be truncated by an artificial boundary [10–12]. Here, we opt for the Sommerfeld boundary condition and hence, the problem reads:

$$\begin{cases} -\omega^2 y - \nabla \cdot (u\nabla y) = f, & \text{in } \Omega, \\ \dfrac{\partial y}{\partial n} - iky = 0, & \text{on } \Gamma = \partial\Omega, \end{cases} \tag{5}$$

where $k(x) = \omega/\sqrt{u(x)}$ is the wavenumber at time frequency $\omega$.

The discretization of the continuous problem (5) yields a problem with a finite number of unknowns and here, for the sake of run-time, we opt for a finite difference (FD) method with staggered grid. In the discretized problem, we get a linear system for the forward problem:

$$A(u)\,y = f, \tag{6}$$

where the matrix $A$ corresponds to the Helmholtz problem. By using (6) as the PDE constraint in (2) instead of the time dependent counterpart (1), we avoid large-scale time-dependent data.

According to [2], cutting different kind of tissue with a laser beam produces different range of frequencies, i.e. different spectra. Hence, we may know when the laser starts to cut the hard bone from the spectrum. This allows us to reduce the computational domain to the vertical position where the hard bone starts, we define this position as $y_0$. The minimization problem above is strongly non-convex and severely ill-posed and need to be regularized. We opt for regularization by size reduction [13] and hence build $u$ from $K$ distinct functions such that:

$$u(x) = \sum_{m=1}^{K} \beta_m \phi_m(x), \tag{7}$$

where $\beta_m \in \mathbb{R}$ and $\phi_m$ are defined by:

$$\phi_m(x) = \begin{cases} 1, & \text{for } y_0\left(1 - \dfrac{m}{K}\right) < x_2 \leq y_0\left(1 - \dfrac{m-1}{K}\right), \\ 0, & \text{otherwise.} \end{cases} \tag{8}$$

Here again, $y_0$ denotes the vertical point from which, we would like to reconstruct the parameter $u$. The parameter $x_2$ denotes the vertical direction of the space variable $x$. In Fig. 1, we illustrate a function $\phi_m$ on a $(0,1) \times (0,1)$ computational domain with $y_0 = 0.7$, $K = 100$ and $m = 50$. By building $u$ as in (7), we use additional information that we are cutting a long bone. The regularization then restricts the solution to reasonable solutions and thus regularizes the optimization problem.

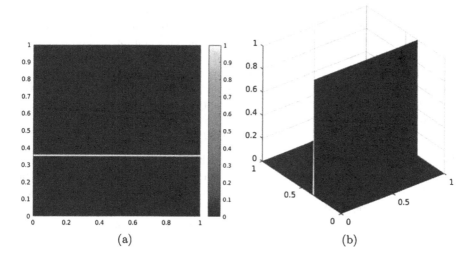

(a)                                    (b)

**Fig. 1.** Illustration of a function $\phi_m$ with $y_0 = 0.7$, $K = 100$ and $m = 50$. (a) Two-dimensional view. (b) Three-dimensional view.

After reducing the dimension of $u$ through (7), we opt for the reduced-space approach. In the reduced-space approach the wave field variable $y$ is eliminated from the objective functional as $\mathcal{F}(u) = \mathcal{F}(y(u), u)$, taking advantage of the linearity of the underlying Helmholtz equation (6) and uniqueness of its solution under appropriate boundary conditions [4]. We can now write the optimization problem (2) as follows:

$$\text{minimize } \mathcal{F}(\beta) = \frac{1}{2} \left\| PA^{-1}(u)f - y^{obs} \right\|_{L^2}^2 , \tag{9}$$

such that $u$ satisfies (7) and $\beta_{min} \leq \beta_m \leq \beta_{max}$ for $m = 1, \ldots, K$. The additional restriction on $\beta_m$ for $m = 1, \ldots, K$ from (7) ensures only reasonable solutions, as $\beta_{min}$ and $\beta_{max}$ are chosen to be the minimal and maximal wave velocities in the body, respectively. To optimize (9), we consider the truncated Gauss-Newton method, using conjugate gradient-iteration with the Eisenstat-Walker criterion [6]. For more details about the parameters chosen for the truncated Newton method we refer to [8].

## 2.2    Method Settings

To perform a bone cut with a laser, a high power pulsed laser is used. Acoustic waves with higher frequencies are produced when cutting cortical bones; and lower frequencies when cutting muscles or other soft tissues [2]. This difference in the frequencies, is a key point in reconstructing the bone structure and for an accurate depth control.

In Fig. 2, we show a typical long bone structure with soft tissue, cortical hard bone and bone marrow and consider a slice of it in the area of 10 mm × 10 mm. At the top of Fig. 2, we illustrate the tip of the laser together with a bone structure with different tissues and their respective wave velocities: the first layer is a muscle with wave velocity of $v = 1568$ m/s, the second is a hard bone (cortical) with wave velocity of $v = 4080$ m/s, the third layer consist of bone marrow with wave velocity of $v = 1700$ m/s. The next layer is once again a hard bone and right after there is soft tissue on the posterior side, which might contain nerves or blood vessels. To illustrate the inhomogeneity of the tissue, we set the squared medium velocity as:

$$u = v^2(1 + 0.01\xi), \tag{10}$$

where $v$ is the respective wave velocity of each tissue and $\xi$ is a standard i.i.d. random variable with mean zero and variance equal to one. The two stars on the top of Fig. 2 represent the location of the two microphones recording the wave produced by the bone ablation process. To avoid inverse crime, i.e. a situation when the same (or very nearly the same) theoretical ingredients are employed to

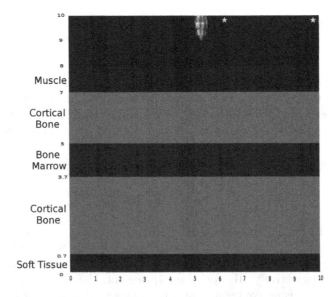

**Fig. 2.** Method settings: a laser beam is ready to cut through several layers of tissues with different wave velocities. The locations of the microphones recording the acoustic waves are indicated with green stars at the top of the figure. (Color figure online)

synthesize as well as to invert data in an inverse problem [14], the measurements on the true profile were computed on a finer different mesh which is not coupled with the computational mesh. Furthermore, we add to the measurements 10% of standard Gaussian noise, s.t.:

$$y^{obs} = \hat{y}^{obs}(1 + 0.1\xi), \tag{11}$$

where $\hat{y}^{obs}$ is the measurements without added noise and $\xi$ is a standard i.i.d. random variable with mean zero and variance equal to one.

## 3   Results

Since we can differentiate between the spectra of the bone and the muscle, we may start our computation at the point where the laser cuts through the muscle and reach the bone for the first time. The true profile is shown in Fig. 3(c). At this point a wave with high frequency is produced and we assume that its frequency is equal to 0.2 MHz [2]. In Fig. 3(b), we illustrate the real part of the wave $y$ propagating through the true medium in the 10 mm × 10 mm domain. Hence, we set $y_0$ from (8) to 7 mm, the vertical position where the hard bone starts and our initial start value for the medium $u$ is shown in Fig. 3(a).

Now, we solve (9) on a relatively coarse finite-difference grid, i.e. 100 × 100, for fast computation (our goal is to get results which can deliver live feedback during the laser ablation). We get an accurate reconstruction of the exact depth, where each one of the first two layers (upper cortical and marrow bone) begins and ends, see Fig. 3(d).

Yet, the reconstruction does not hold enough accurate information on the second layer of the cortical bone. The reconstruction of the second layer is very critical as nerves or blood vessels might be behind it. At this point, we need to reconstruct not only the second layer of the cortical bone, but also the position of the cut. Again, we use the same microphones positions, to know when the laser beam reached the second layer of the hard bone after cutting through the marrow (that means significantly higher frequency). At this point, we use the information on the first two bone-layers of the result, shown in Fig. 3(d), as the new initial value for $u$. Now, we are not only opt for the full bone structure represented by $u$, but also for the depth, represented by $x_2$, of the source $f(x_1, x_2)$. Hence, we write a new optimization problem:

$$\text{minimize } \mathcal{F}(u, x_2) = \frac{1}{2} \left\| PA^{-1}(u)f(x_1, x_2) - y^{obs} \right\|_{L^2}^2. \tag{12}$$

Note that, the optimal $x_2$ changes not only the source $f$, but the medium $u$ as well, since the bone above the point $x_2$ has already been cut. This makes this optimization problem a mixture between optimal control, where we look for the properties of the source and inverse medium problem, where we look for the properties of the medium. Again, we use the same setup as above for solving (12).

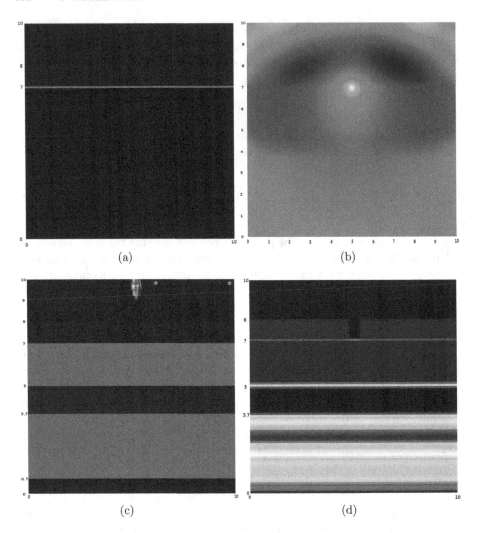

**Fig. 3.** Reconstruction of the two first layers of the bone. (a) The initial value for $u$. (b) The acoustic wave in the frequency domain propagating through the true medium. (c) The true profile just after cutting through the muscle. (d) The reconstruction of the first hard bone and the bone marrow.

We can solve (12) at several time-points during the ablation of the second layer of the cortical bone to get a control on the depth to give feedback to the surgeon during the cut of this critical stage of the cut. Here, we solve (12) in two critical points: first, when starting to cut the second cortical bone and second, which is the most critical one, is when cutting through the bone. On the top-left of Fig. 4, we show the true bone structure together with the true position of the cut $(5, 3.7)$. At the top-right of Fig. 4, we display the reconstruction of $u$ together with the detection of the position of the source. The reconstructed

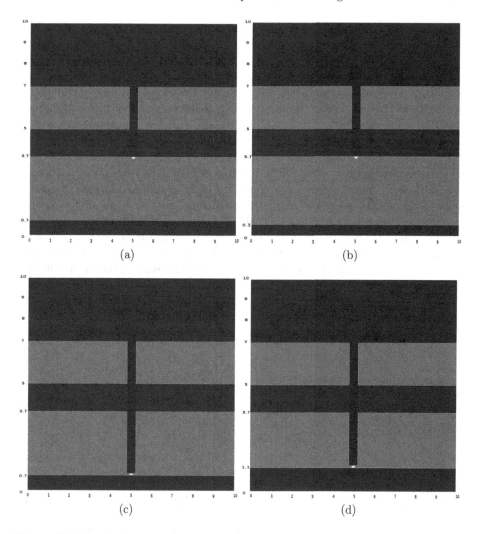

**Fig. 4.** Finding both true position of the cut and the second layer of the cortical bone. (a), (c) The true profiles with the true positions of the cut. (b), (d) The final reconstructions of $u$ and the depth $x_2$ from the solution of (12).

source position $(5, 3.7)$ is accurate and the reconstruction of the last layer of $u$ ends at $x_2 = 0.5$ mm instead of at $x_2 = 0.7$ mm in the true profile (error of 0.2 mm). At the bottom-left of Fig. 4, we display the true structure of the bone, this time the position of the true cut is at $(5, 0.7)$. The reconstructed source position is at $(5, 1.1)$, which is 0.4 mm away from the true cut position. However, the end of the reconstructed second layer of the cortical bone ends at 1.1 as well and hence, the reconstruction implies that the laser beam has been cut through the bone and no further laser cut is allowed. This detection of the end of the layer is, likely, because of the strong reflection of the wave when cutting at the end of the layer. Hence, the method successfully detected the point when the laser beam was cutting through the whole bone.

Even if the solution is dependent in the noise, in our simulations, a typical error was not exceeding the 0.4 mm, which shows a good stability for the method, even when using only two microphones. An additional way to reduce the sensitivity of the solution to the noise is to increase the number of microphones.

## 4  Conclusions

This paper gives a framework for performing depth control when cutting bones with laser. We adapt the inverse medium problem to the medical use of a laser beam to get control of the cutting-depth and hence, may prevent collateral damage on blood vessels, nerves or other soft tissues around the bones being cut.

These initial results show that depth control using the acoustic waves produced during laser ablation is in theory possible and yet, we have to use real data to quantify how accurate the acoustic waves enable for solving the inverse media problem, especially in three space dimensions. The expansion of the inverse problem from two-dimensional to three-dimensional has been done before in geophysical exploration, without major changes in the algorithms, see for example [15]. The method can be extended to any kind of bone-shape using the adaptive eigenspace [8].

**Acknowledgements.** This work has been part of the MIRACLE Project funded by the Werner Siemens Foundation, Zug/Switzerland.

## References

1. Burgner, J., Müller, M., Raczkowsky, J., Wörn, H.: Ex vivo accuracy evaluation for robot assisted laser bone ablation. Int. J. Med. Robot. **6**(4), 489–500 (2010). https://doi.org/10.1002/rcs.366
2. Nguendon, H., et al.: Characterization of ablated porcine bone and muscle using laser-induced acoustic wave method for tissue differentiation. In: Lilge, L. (ed.) Proceedings of European Conferences on Biomedical Optics, Medical Laser Applications and Laser-Tissue Interactions VIII, vol. 10417, p. 104170N. SPIE (2017). https://doi.org/0.1117/12.2286121
3. Nahum, U.: Adaptive eigenspace for inverse problems in the frequency domain. Ph.D. thesis, University of Basel, Switzerland (2016)
4. Haber, E., Ascher, U., Oldenburg, D.: On optimization techniques for solving nonlinear inverse problems. Inverse Probl. **16**(5), 1263 (2000). https://doi.org/10.1088/0266-5611/16/5/309
5. Nash, S.: A survey of truncated-Newton methods. J. Comput. Appl. Math. **124**(1–2), 45–59 (2000). https://doi.org/10.1016/S0377-0427(00)00426-X
6. Eisenstat, S., Walker, H.: Choosing the forcing terms in an inexact Newton method. SIAM J. Sci. Comput. **17**(1), 16–32 (1996). https://doi.org/10.1137/0917003
7. Métivier, L., Bretaudeau, F., Brossier, R., Operto, S., Virieux, J.: Full waveform inversion and the truncated Newton method: quantitative imaging of complex subsurface structures. Geophys. Prospect. **62**(6), 1353–1375 (2014). https://doi.org/10.1111/1365-2478.12136

8. Grote, M., Kraym, M., Nahum, U.: Adaptive eigenspace method for inverse scattering problems in the frequency domain. Inverse Probl. **33**(2), 025006 (2017). https://doi.org/10.1088/1361-6420/aa5250

9. de Buhan, M., Kray, M.: A new approach to solve the inverse scattering problem for waves: combining the TRAC and the adaptive inversion methods. Inverse Probl. **29**(8), 085009 (2013). https://doi.org/10.1088/0266-5611/29/8/085009

10. Bayliss, A., Turkel, E.: Radiation boundary conditions for wave-like equations. Comm. Pure Appl. Math. **33**(6), 707–725 (1980). https://doi.org/10.1002/cpa.3160330603

11. Engquist, B., Majda, A.: Absorbing boundary conditions for the numerical simulation of waves. Math. Comput. **31**(139), 629–651 (1977). https://doi.org/10.1073/pnas.74.5.1765

12. Grote, M., Keller, J.: Nonreflecting boundary conditions for time-dependent scattering. J. Comput. Phys. **127**(1), 52–65 (1996). https://doi.org/10.1006/jcph.1996.0157

13. Chavent, G.: Nonlinear Least Squares for Inverse Problems. Springer, Heidelberg (1996). https://doi.org/10.1007/978-90-481-2785-6

14. Wirgin, A.: The inverse crime. arXiv:math-ph/0401050 (2004)

15. Operto, S., et al.: Efficient 3-D frequency-domain mono-parameter full-waveform inversion of ocean-bottom cable data: application to Valhall in the visco-acoustic vertical transverse isotropic approximation. Geophys. J. Int. **202**(2), 1362–1391 (2015). https://doi.org/10.1093/gji/ggv226

# Automated Dynamic 3D Ultrasound Assessment of Developmental Dysplasia of the Infant Hip

Olivia Paserin[1]([✉]), Kishore Mulpuri[2], Anthony Cooper[2], Antony J. Hodgson[3], and Rafeef Garbi[1]

[1] Department of Electrical and Computer Engineering,
University of British Columbia, Vancouver, Canada
opaserin@ece.ubc.ca
[2] Department of Orthopaedic Surgery, British Columbia Children's Hospital,
Vancouver, Canada
[3] Department of Mechanical Engineering,
University of British Columbia, Vancouver, Canada

**Abstract.** Dynamic two-dimensional sonography of the infant hip is a commonly used procedure for developmental dysplasia of the hip (DDH) screening by many clinicians. It however has been found to be unreliable with some studies reporting associated misdiagnosis rates of up to 29%. Aiming to improve reliability of diagnosis and to help in standardizing diagnosis across different raters and health-centers, we present a preliminary automated method for assessing hip instability using three-dimensional (3D) dynamic ultrasound (US). To quantify hip assessment, we propose the use of femoral head coverage variability ($\Delta FHC_{3D}$) within US volumes collected during a dynamic scan which uses phase symmetry features to approximate the vertical cortex of the ilium and a random forest classifier to identify the approximate location of the femoral head. We measure the change in $FHC_{3D}$ across US scans of the hip acquired under posterior stress vs. rest as maneuvered during a 3D dynamic assessment. Our findings on 38 hips from 19 infants scanned by one orthopedic surgeon and two radiology technicians suggests the proposed $\Delta FHC_{3D}$ may provide a good degree of repeatability with an average test-retest intraclass correlation measure of 0.70 (95% confidence interval: 0.35 to 0.87, $F(21, 21) = 7.738$, $p < 0.001$). This suggests that our 3D dynamic dysplasia metric may prove valuable in improving reliability in diagnosing hip laxity due to DDH, which may lead to a more standardized DDH assessment with better diagnostic accuracy. The long-term significance of this approach to evaluating dynamic assessments may lie in increasing early diagnostic sensitivity in order to prevent dysplasia remaining undetected prior to manifesting itself in early adulthood joint disease.

**Keywords:** Pediatric · Ultrasound · Hip · Bone imaging
Developmental dysplasia of the hip · DDH · Dynamic assessment
Repeatability

© Springer Nature Switzerland AG 2019
T. Vrtovec et al. (Eds.): MSKI 2018, LNCS 11404, pp. 136–145, 2019.
https://doi.org/10.1007/978-3-030-11166-3_12

# 1    Introduction

Performing dynamic sonography on the infant hip is a routine part of screening for developmental dysplasia of the hip (DDH) in many clinical settings [1]. However, such screening has been shown to be unreliable. For example, in a study on a cohort of 266 infants by Imrie et al. [2]., dynamic assessment was associated with misdiagnosis rates of 29% where infants who had been screened as healthy were later found to display sufficient signs of dysplasia to require treatment In a dynamic assessment of an infant's hip, clinicians apply stress to the adducted hip, in a posterior direction to provoke dislocation, and observe the resulting joint movement with ultrasound (US) [3]. Barlow (dislocation) and Ortolani (reduction) maneuvers have become the basis for the clinical classification of hip abnormality [3]. Resulting observations are currently described qualitatively using terms such as normal, lax, dislocatable, reducible and not reducible, and are not based on measured quantities. Evaluating the hip's stability dynamically is crucial because in order to avoid DDH, the development of the neonatal cartilaginous acetabulum must occur around *"a properly seated femoral head"* [4]. In a complementary manner, Graf's method [5] is the standardized method for assessing acetabular morphology of the infant hip using US-based angle measurements to estimate the depth of the acetabular socket during a static assessment. However, characterizing acetabular morphology with Graf's technique alone does not evaluate or screen for loose ligaments supporting the hip - a factor in hip dysplasia. As such, dynamic assessment is recommended as a routine part of every infant hip clinical exam [3]. In a recent study by Alamdaran et al. [6]), 100% of hips with dysplastic morphology (mild and severe) were unstable in dynamic analysis while 9% of unstable hips had normal morphology in static evaluation, supporting the need for dynamic assessments to be performed on every hip that appears morphologically normal as they may reduce the number of missed DDH cases [7].

In a recent systematic review, Charlton et al. [8] examined dynamic US screening for hip instability in the first six weeks after birth and found current best practices for such early screening techniques to be still divergent between different institutions in terms of clinical scanning protocols, namely the most appropriate scanning plane and position, diagnostic metrics, patient age to scan, and followup procedures, used internationally. They in fact identified nearly 20 early dynamic US screening techniques present in the literature each with different imaging and measurement protocols. To the best of our knowledge, all previous dynamic assessment studies employed two-dimensional (2D) ultrasonography. However, it has been recently shown that using three-dimensional (3D) US can markedly improve the reliability of dysplasia metric measurements during static assessment of an infant's hip compared to 2D US as volumetric scans can capture the entire hip joint and are less prone to probe orientation errors compared to 2D scans [9,10]. Further, none of the previous dynamic studies explored automating the assessment via computational image analysis despite inter-assessor variability likely accounting for much of the poor reproducibility of dynamic assessments and the related rates of misdiagnosis.

Our main objective in this work is to develop and evaluate an automated quantitative method for assessing hip instability volumetrically in a dynamic examination in order to improve reliability of diagnosis and reduce misdiagnosis rates. To enable this, we developed an approach to automatically calculate femoral head coverage ($FHC_{3D}$) from volumetric US scans, a ratio describing how much of the femoral head sits in the acetabular cup of the hip joint [11]. While the intra-rater variability of automatic $FHC_{3D}$ measurements in static assessments was found to be 5.4% and the inter-rater variability to be 6.1% [11], the variability of the measurement during dynamic assessment it is not yet known, nor is the range of differences in $FHC_{3D}$ during dynamic evaluations across normal and dysplastic hips. In an initial feasibility study [12] we recently used our automatic $FHC_{3D}$ measurement technique to perform a dynamic assessment on a single patient, but this protocol did not include a repeated measurement. In this paper, therefore, we report on a clinical study evaluating the test-retest repeatability of an automatic technique for estimating *change* in $FHC_{3D}$ during dynamic assessments in a larger and more clinically representative cohort of patients. We estimate hip joint laxity by quantifying the change in $FHC_{3D}$ observed during a dynamic assessment as the hip is posteriorly stressed by a clinician. With stress applied to a stable joint, we expect femoral head coverage to vary minimally while an unstable hip would show larger changes in the measurement during distraction.

## 2    Materials and Method

### 2.1    Data Acquisition and Experimental Setup

In this study, one pediatric orthopedic surgeon and two technologists from the radiology department at British Columbia Children's Hospital participated in collecting B-mode 3D US images of 38 infant hips from 19 patients. All patients had been referred to the orthopedic clinic due to DDH risk factors and/or clinical suspicion for DDH in one or both hips. Patient inclusion criteria included being between the ages of 0–4 months and attending an appointment for suspected or confirmed DDH. The principal exclusion criterion was that subjects had not received a diagnosis of a genetic syndrome, since patients with genetic syndromes often have abnormal hips due to non DDH-related conditions and we wanted to eliminate that as a potential confounder. Parents were informed of our research goals and protocols, as well as their right to withdraw their consent at any time during the imaging procedure without affecting their child's clinical care. Age at scan, sex, born by caesarian section, breech birth position, and birth order patient demographics were recorded and are summarized in Table 1. 79% of the patients were female. Interestingly, the majority (68%) of referred patients were first born and had no familial history of DDH.

3D US volumes were obtained as part of routine clinical care under appropriate institutional review board approval. Data collection for our study coincided with patients' regular clinic visit and increased each appointment duration by approximately five minutes. 3D US volumes were collected using a SonixTouch

**Table 1.** Summary demographics of our 19 patient cohort, including developmental dysplasia of the hip risk factors.

| Patient demographics in our clinical study | |
|---|---|
| Age | 0 to 4 months |
| Sex | 14 female; 5 male |
| Affected hip | 8 left; 5 right; 6 bilateral |
| Familial history of DDH | 3 yes; 13 no; 3 unknown |
| First born child | 13 yes; 6 no |
| Breech presentation | 11 yes; 8 no |
| Caesarian section | 11 yes; 8 no |

Q+ scanner (BK ultrasound, Analogic Inc., Peabody, MA, USA) with a 4DL14-5/38 linear 4D transducer set at 7 MHz. The probe was held laterally and positioned in the coronal plane with the infant laying on their side with their hip flexed. Each acquired volume comprised 245 slices with an axial resolution of 0.17 mm and an in-plane resolution of $256 \times 256$ pixels corresponding to a physical slice dimension of $38 \times 38$ mm.

To investigate test-retest repeatability, each hip examination involved two dynamic assessments performed by one rater (out of the three participating sonographers). The pediatric orthopaedic surgeon, first radiology technologist, and second radiology technologist performed the assessment on twelve, three, and four of the 19 patients, respectively. Each dynamic assessment involved acquiring two 3D US volumes - one with and one without stress applied to the joint in an effort to observe maximal displacement (i.e. we acquired four 3D US volumes for each hip and eight 3D US volumes in total for each patient). We did not evaluate inter-rater repeatability due to the additional time that would have been required from attending clinical staff and families for each patient visit.

### 2.2   Identifying Adequate Volumes

In order to evaluate test-retest repeatability, we required all four volumes (test neutral, test stressed, retest neutral, retest stressed) from each hip to be adequate for interpretation as in [13]. Volumes were independently classified as adequate vs. inadequate using the deep learning-based classifier presented in [13] found to perform with 82% accuracy compared with an expert radiologist's labels as ground truth. The classifier was comprised of five convolutional layers to extract hierarchical features from a scan, followed by a recurrent, long short-term memory layer to capture the spatial relationship of their responses.

### 2.3   Femoral Head and Ilium Segmentation

To automatically estimate $FHC_{3D}$ in each US volume, we used the method proposed by [11]. Before segmenting anatomical structures, we first extracted a 3D bone boundary of the hip joint using a rotation-invariant local symmetry feature, structured phase symmetry, which extracts sheet-like hyperechoic responses in the volume including bone boundaries, cartilage boundaries, and soft tissue interfaces [14]. The bone boundaries were isolated using attenuation-based post-processing.

From the extracted bone boundaries, we next identified a planar approximation to the vertical cortex of the ilium using geometric priors and a M-estimator sample consensus (MSAC) algorithm [15]. Next, we extracted a voxel-wise probability map characterizing the likelihood of a voxel belonging to the femoral head, a hypoechoic spherical structure localized with a trained random forest classifier.

Once both the ilium and femoral head were segmented, we then used both these structures to calculate $FHC_{3D}$ as the ratio of femoral head portion medial to plane of the ilium as illustrated in Fig. 1. Finally, we estimate the joint laxity by computing $\Delta FHC_{3D} = FHC_{neutral} - FHC_{stressed}$ where $FHC_{neutral}$ was measured from the volume in which no stress was applied and $FHC_{stressed}$ was measured from the volume in which the clinician applied stress in a direction posterior to the hip joint.

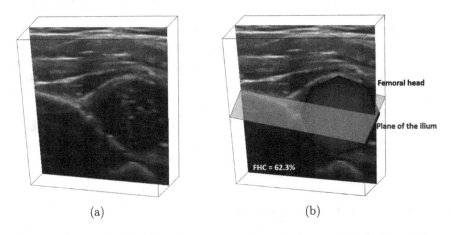

(a)                                    (b)

**Fig. 1.** (a) Three-dimensional visualization of the raw ultrasound (US) data with one coronal slice from the volume displayed. (b) Overlay of the example US volume and its automatically extracted femoral head and planar ilium.

## 2.4   Quantifying Joint Laxity

Our proposed $FHC_{3D}$ ratio is again illustrated in Fig. 2; $FHC_{3D}$ was calculated as the ratio of the femoral head portion medial to the plane of the ilium. Examples of both unstable and stable hips are shown. With stress applied to a stable hip joint, we expect $FHC_{3D}$ to vary minimally. On the other hand, an unstable hip would show large changes in $FHC_{3D}$ as the femoral head does not sit well in the acetabular socket. Hence, we used $\Delta FHC_{3D}$ to quantify joint stability, where $\Delta FHC_{3D} = FHC_{neutral} - FHC_{stressed}$.

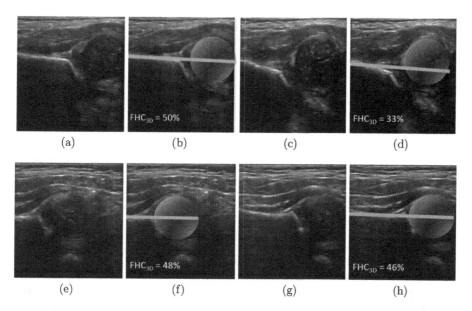

**Fig. 2.** Qualitative results. (a)–(d) Hip demonstrating 17% change in $FHC_{3D}$. (a) Raw ultrasound (US) volume with hip at rest. (b) Overlay of the femoral head and planar ilium segmentations. (c) Raw US volume with the hip stressed posteriorly. (a) Overlay of the femoral head and planar ilium segmentations. (e)–(h) Hip demonstrating 2% change in $FHC_{3D}$. (e) Raw US volume with hip at rest. (f) Overlay of the femoral head and planar ilium segmentations. (g) Raw US volume with the hip stressed posteriorly. (h) Overlay of the femoral head and planar ilium segmentations.

## 3   Results and Discussion

Our resulting $FHC_{3D}$ and $\alpha_{3D}$ from all recorded repeated dynamic assessments are plotted in Figs. 3 and 4. In post-clinical visit analysis, half of our dynamic assessment recordings were found to have had one or more of the four volumes classified as inadequate, which demonstrates that, despite the increased viewing volumes that 3D scan provide, it is nonetheless still difficult for clinicians to reliably acquire high quality 3D US volumes. We found that most inadequate volumes were acquired during sessions where a new sonographer was collecting the data, which suggests that additional training in operating the 3D US probe may be required. This left us with seventeen test-retest assessments that had all four required dynamic volumes successfully classified as adequate; these were therefore included in the statistical analysis below.

High test-retest repeatability is a necessary requirement for demonstrating the utility of a quantified dynamic assessment diagnostic tool. Using the well-established intra-class correlation coefficient (ICC) performance measures [16], we quantify the reliability of the dynamic assessment done with 3D US. A good degree of reliability was found between the measurements. The test-retest

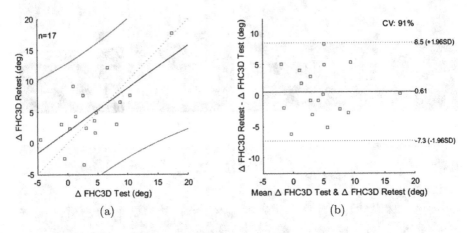

**Fig. 3.** $FHC_{3D}$ measurements and Bland-Altman plot ($\Delta FHC_{3D}$ repeatability). (a) Scatter plot of test-retest $FHC_{3D}$ measurements. Every dot represents two measurements acquired by one rater for one hip. Solid line shows line of best fit and dotted line shows 1−1 line. Curved lines show fit line confidence intervals. (b) Bland-Altman plot for test-retest $FHC_{3D}$ measurements. The solid line indicates the mean difference ($M = 0.61$), dashed lines mark mean difference $\pm 1.96$ standard deviations (SDs). $SD = 4.05$. CV is coefficient of variation (SD of mean values as a percentage).

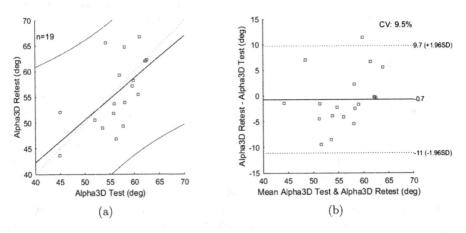

**Fig. 4.** $\alpha_{3D}$ measurements and Bland-Altman plot ($\alpha_{3D}$ repeatability). (a) Scatter plot of test-retest $\alpha_{3D}$ measurements. Every point represents two measurements acquired by one rater for one hip. Solid line shows line of best fit and dotted line shows 1−1 line. Curved lines show fit line confidence intervals. (b) Bland-Altman plot for test-retest $\alpha_{3D}$ measurements. The solid line indicates the mean difference ($M = -0.70$), dashed lines mark mean difference $\pm 1.96$ standard deviations (SDs). $SD = 5.33$. CV is coefficient of variation (SD of mean values as a percentage).

ICC measure of 0.70 (95% confidence interval: 0.35 to 0.87, $F(21, 21) = 7.738$, $p < 0.001$). ICC estimates and their 95% confident intervals were calculated using MATLAB (Mathworks Inc., Natick, MA, USA) based on a single measurement, absolute-agreement, 2-way mixed-effects model. As shown in Fig. 3, mean difference of $\Delta FHC_{3D}$ measurements was 0.61 with standard deviation (SD) 4.05. This suggests that the proposed metric and technique likely have sufficient resolution and repeatability to quantify differences in laxity between stable and mildly unstable hips, since the observed changes in $\Delta FHC_{3D}$ range up to about 18% in this cohort. Due to the unbalanced number of volumes recorded by each observer, we have not included their results separately, however this comparison analysis will be performed and reported in future work once we acquire a larger dataset.

Additionally, we automatically computed the $\alpha_{3D}$ measurements on each hip and measured a test-retest ICC measure of 0.61 (95% confidence interval: 0.22 to 0.83, ($F(18, 18) = 4.05$, $p < 0.01$) for $\alpha_{3D}$. This calculation was also based on a single measurement, absolute-agreement, 2-way mixed-effects model. As shown in Fig. 4, mean difference of repeated $\alpha_{3D}$ measurements was 0.70 with SD 5.33. We found that the most unstable hip, as determined by $\Delta FHC_{3D}$ with a change of 17% during the dynamic assessment, corresponded to the most dysplastic hip, as determined by $\alpha_{3D}$ with an angle of less than 40°, demonstrating agreement between the two diagnostic metrics ($\Delta FHC_{3D}$ and $\alpha_{3D}$) in that case. In future work, we plan to collect more US-recorded dynamic assessments in order to determine a reliable range of $\Delta FHC_{3D}$ for both stable and dysplastic infant hips.

**Computation Complexity.** The process of segmenting one US volume and extracting $FHC_{3D}$ took approximately 100 seconds when run on a Intel (R) Xeon(R) 3.70 GHz CPU computer with 8 GB RAM. All processes were executed using MATLAB 2018a. Current practice has a sonographer process the images post-acquisition, so this computation time is not a significant barrier to implementation as it is not necessary to deliver the head coverage metric in near-real time. Nonetheless, although not critical for clinical use, we plan to work towards optimizing our code with graphics processing unit (GPU) parallel programming to significantly reduce this computation time. Volume adequacy classification was performed in one second per volume, a time suitable for clinical workflow, although this was not implemented in near-real time in this study, but was performed post-facto. This time was achieved on a Intel(R) Core(TM) i7-7800X 3.50 GHz CPU, with a NVIDIA TITAN Xp GPU and 64 GB of RAM.

## 4    Conclusions

We presented an automatic 3D dysplasia metric, $\Delta FHC_{3D}$, to characterize DDH from 3D US images of the neonatal hip through a 3D dynamic assessment procedure. In previous studies [9], $\alpha_{3D}$ was reported to have an intra-rater reliability of 2.2° ($p < 0.01$) and an inter-rater reliability of 2.35° ($p < 0.01$). We suspect that the observed increase in variability in our study was due to the increased amount of movement introduced during dynamic assessment, as the values reported in [9] were acquired during static assessments only. Mean difference of $\Delta FHC_{3D}$ measurements was 0.61 with SD 4.05, with $\Delta FHC_{3D}$ values ranging from 0 to 17%. Using the proposed $\Delta FHC_{3D}$ we achieved a good degree of reliability. This suggests that this 3D dynamic dysplasia metric could be valuable in improving the reliability in diagnosing hip laxity due to DDH, which may lead to a more standardized DDH assessment with better diagnostic accuracy.

**Acknowledgements.** We gratefully acknowledge the support of NVIDIA Corporation with the donation of the Titan X GPU used for this research.

# References

1. Bracken, J., Ditchfield, M.: Ultrasonography in developmental dysplasia of the hip: what have we learned? Pediatr. Radiol. **42**(12), 1418–1431 (2012). https://doi.org/10.1007/s00247-012-2429-8
2. Imrie, M., Scott, V., Stearns, P., Bastrom, T., Mubarak, S.: Is ultrasound screening for DDH in babies born breech sufficient? J. Child. Orthop. **4**(1), 3–8 (2010). https://doi.org/10.1007/s11832-009-0217-2
3. Harcke, H., Grissom, L.: Performing dynamic sonography of the infant hip. AJR Am. J. Roentgenol. **155**(4), 837–844 (1990). https://doi.org/10.2214/ajr.155.4.2119119
4. Gomes, H., Ouedraogo, T., Avisse, C., Lallemand, A., Bakhache, P.: Neonatal hip: from anatomy to cost-effective sonography. Eur. Radiol. **8**(6), 1030–1039 (1998). https://doi.org/10.1007/s003300050510
5. Graf, R.: New possibilities for the diagnosis of congenital hip joint dislocation by ultrasonography. J. Pediatr. Orthop. **3**(3), 354–359 (1983)
6. Alamdaran, S., Kazemi, S., Parsa, A., Moghadam, M., Feyzi, A., Mardani, R.: Assessment of diagnostic value of single view dynamic technique in diagnosis of developmental dysplasia of hip: a comparison with static and dynamic ultrasound techniques. Arch. Bone Joint Surg. **4**(4), 371–375 (2016)
7. Koşar, P., Ergun, E., Unlübay, D., Koşar, U.: Comparison of morphologic and dynamic US methods in examination of the newborn hip. Diagn. Interv. Radiol. **15**(4), 284–289 (2009). https://doi.org/10.4261/1305-3825.DIR.2557-09.2
8. Charlton, S., Schoo, A., Walters, L.: Early dynamic ultrasound for neonatal hip instability: implications for rural Australia. BMC Pediatr. **17**, 82 (2017). https://doi.org/10.1186/s12887-017-0830-z
9. Quader, N., Hodgson, A., Mulpuri, K., Cooper, A., Abugharbieh, R.: Towards reliable automatic characterization of neonatal hip dysplasia from 3D ultrasound images. In: Ourselin, S., Joskowicz, L., Sabuncu, M.R., Unal, G., Wells, W. (eds.) MICCAI 2016. LNCS, vol. 9900, pp. 602–609. Springer, Cham (2016). https://doi.org/10.1007/978-3-319-46720-7_70
10. Jaremko, J., Mabee, M., Swami, V., Jamieson, L., Chow, K., Thompson, R.: Potential for change in US diagnosis of hip dysplasia solely caused by changes in probe orientation: patterns of alpha-angle variation revealed by using three-dimensional US. Radiology **273**(3), 870–878 (2014). https://doi.org/10.1148/radiol.14140451

11. Quader, N., Hodgson, A.J., Mulpuri, K., Cooper, A., Abugharbieh, R.: A 3D femoral head coverage metric for enhanced reliability in diagnosing hip dysplasia. In: Descoteaux, M., Maier-Hein, L., Franz, A., Jannin, P., Collins, D.L., Duchesne, S. (eds.) MICCAI 2017. LNCS, vol. 10433, pp. 100–107. Springer, Cham (2017). https://doi.org/10.1007/978-3-319-66182-7_12

12. Paserin, O., Mulpuri, K., Cooper, A., Abugharbieh, R., Hodgson, A.: Improving 3D ultrasound scan adequacy classification using a three-slice convolutional neural network architecture. In: Zhan, W., Rodriguez Y Baena, F. (eds.) Proceedings of Annual Meeting of the International Society for Computer Assisted Orthopaedic Surgery - CAOS 2018, EPiC Series in Health Sciences, vol. 2, pp. 152–156 (2018). https://doi.org/10.29007/2tct

13. Paserin, O., Mulpuri, K., Cooper, A., Hodgson, A.J., Garbi, R.: Real time RNN based 3D ultrasound scan adequacy for developmental dysplasia of the hip. In: Frangi, A.F., Schnabel, J.A., Davatzikos, C., Alberola-López, C., Fichtinger, G. (eds.) MICCAI 2018. LNCS, vol. 11070, pp. 365–373. Springer, Cham (2018). https://doi.org/10.1007/978-3-030-00928-1_42

14. Quader, N., Hodgson, A., Abugharbieh, R.: Confidence weighted local phase features for robust bone surface segmentation in ultrasound. In: Linguraru, M.G., et al. (eds.) CLIP 2014. LNCS, vol. 8680, pp. 76–83. Springer, Cham (2014). https://doi.org/10.1007/978-3-319-13909-8_10

15. Torr, P., Zisserman, A.: MLESAC: a new robust estimator with application to estimating image geometry. Comput. Vis. Image Underst. **78**(1), 138–156 (2000). https://doi.org/10.1006/cviu.1999.0832

16. McGraw, K., Wong, S.: Forming inferences about some intraclass correlation coefficients. Psychol. Methods **1**(1), 30–46 (1996). https://doi.org/10.1037/1082-989X.1.1.30

# Automated Measurement of Pelvic Incidence from X-Ray Images

Robert Korez[1], Michael Putzier[2], and Tomaž Vrtovec[1(✉)]

[1] Faculty of Electrical Engineering, University of Ljubljana, Ljubljana, Slovenia
tomaz.vrtovec@fe.uni-lj.si
[2] Charité University Hospital, Berlin, Germany

**Abstract.** One of the most important parameters of sagittal pelvic alignment is the pelvic incidence (PI), which is commonly measured from sagittal X-ray images of the pelvis as the angle between the line connecting the midpoint of the femoral head centers with the center of the sacral endplate, and the line orthogonal to the sacral endplate. In this paper, we present the results of a fully automated measurement of PI from X-ray images that is based on the deep learning technologies. In each sagittal X-ray image of the pelvis, regions of interest (sacral endplate and both femoral heads) are first automatically defined, and then landmarks are detected within these regions, i.e. the anterior edge, the center and the posterior edge of the sacral endplate that define the line of the sacral endplate inclination, and the centers of both femoral heads with the corresponding midpoint representing the hip axis. From the hip axis, and the line along the sacral endplate and its center, PI is computed. Measurements were performed on X-ray pelvic images from 38 subjects (15 males/23 females; mean age 71.1 years), and statistical analysis of reference manual and fully automated measurements revealed a relatively good agreement, with the mean absolute difference $\pm$ standard deviation of $5.1 \pm 4.4°$ and Pearson correlation coefficient of $R = 0.82$ ($p$-value below $10^{-6}$), with the paired $t$-test revealing no statistically significant differences ($p$-value above 0.05). The differences between reference manual and fully automated measurements were within the repeatability and reliability of manual measurements, indicating that PI can be accurately determined by the proposed fully automated approach.

**Keywords:** Pelvic incidence · X-ray imaging · Deep learning

## 1 Introduction

Pelvic incidence (PI) is one of the most important parameters of sagittal pelvic alignment, and is represented by the angle between the line connecting the hip axis (i.e. the midpoint of the centers of both femoral heads) with the center of the sacral endplate, and the line orthogonal to the sacral endplate [1,2]. As such, it describes the relative position of the sacral endplate against the femoral heads, and therefore the anatomical characteristics of the pelvis in the sagittal plane

© Springer Nature Switzerland AG 2019
T. Vrtovec et al. (Eds.): MSKI 2018, LNCS 11404, pp. 146–152, 2019.
https://doi.org/10.1007/978-3-030-11166-3_13

and the balance of the lumbar spine that rests on the sacrum. The mean PI for a healthy population is $47°-57°$ with a standard deviation (SD) of around $10°$ [2], nevertheless, a very low PI ($35°-44°$) means that the femoral heads are positioned just below the sacral endplate with the pelvis being narrow horizontally and large vertically (i.e. a vertical pelvis), while a very high PI ($75°-85°$) means that the femoral heads are position ahead of the midpoint of the sacral endplate with the pelvis being narrow vertically and large horizontally (i.e. a horizontal pelvis) [3]. Measurement of PI is most commonly performed in sagittal X-ray images of the pelvis (Fig. 1), however, it represents a relatively tedious and subjective task, mostly because of the quality of the acquired images and their projective nature [4–6]. Although several software packages exist for computerized measurement of PI [4,7–10], the resulting measurements are still based on manually defined points, geometrical constructs and statistical modeling, and therefore are not fully automated. In this paper, we present the results of a fully automated measurement of PI from X-ray images of the pelvis.

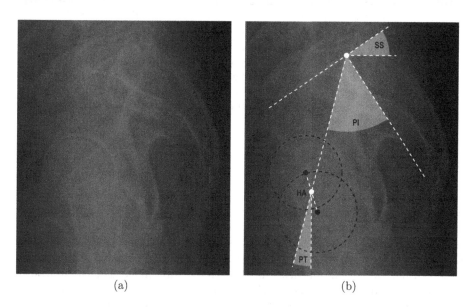

(a)                                      (b)

**Fig. 1.** (a) A sagittal X-ray of the pelvis. (b) The parameters of the pelvic incidence (PI) as the angle between the line connecting the hip axis (HA, the midpoint between the centers of both femoral heads) with the first sacral (S1) endplate center and the line orthogonal to the S1 endplate, sacral slope (SS) as the angle between the line along the S1 endplate and the horizontal reference, and pelvic tilt (PT) as the angle between the line connecting the HA with the S1 endplate center and the vertical reference. The following relationship is established: SS + PT = PI.

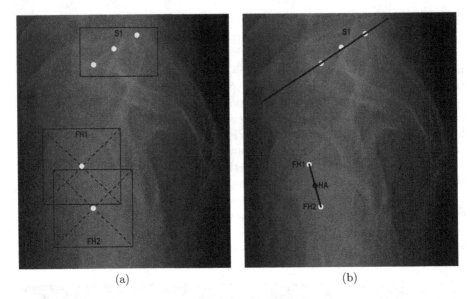

Fig. 2. Fully automated measurement of pelvic incidence. (a) The region of interest (ROI) for the first sacral (S1) endplate and for both femoral heads (FH1, FH2), with landmarks within each ROI: the anterior edge, the center and the posterior edge on the S1 endplate, and the centers of both femoral heads. (b) The sacral slope is determined by fitting a line to the landmarks. The hip axis (HA) is determined as the midpoint between the centers of the femoral heads.

## 2    Methodology

The automated measurement of PI from X-ray pelvic images is based on deep learning and consists of three stages,[1] i.e. the identification of the regions of interest (ROIs), determination of distinctive points or landmarks, and measurement of PI (Fig. 2). The first stage (Fig. 2(a)) is the automated identification of ROIs that contain the observed anatomical structures, i.e. the first sacral (S1) endplate and each individual femoral head, in the given X-ray image. For this purpose, we designed a special architecture of convolutional neural networks (CNNs) [11] that was trained on a set of X-ray images with predefined ROIs. The second stage (Fig. 2(a)) is the automated determination of landmarks, i.e. the center of each femoral head and the anterior edge, the center and the posterior edge of the S1 endplate, within the corresponding ROIs obtained in the first stage. For this purpose, we designed a second CNN architecture [12] that was trained on a set of X-ray images with predefined landmarks. The third stage (Fig. 2(b)) is the automated determination of the line along the S1 endplate, which is obtained by least square fitting to the landmarks defined on the S1 endplate in the second

---

[1] Due to a copyright agreement, we cannot entirely disclose the technical details of our methodology. We therefore invite the reader to focus on the clinical application and the obtained results.

stage, and the determination of the hip axis as the midpoint between the centers of both femoral heads. From the acquired data, we can measure PI as the sum of SS and PT.

## 3   Results

The automated measurement of PI was evaluated on sagittal X-ray images of the pelvis from 44 subjects (16 males/28 females; mean age 71.5 years, age range 49–85 years) that were acquired at Charité University Hospital (Berlin, Germany) by the Kodak Elite CR and Kodak DRX-Evolution scanners (Carestream Health; Rochester, New York, USA) for purposes not related to this retrospective study. For each image, reference manual measurements of PI, SS and PT were obtained, which allowed for a statistical comparison with the fully automated measurements. However, reference manual measurements could not be reliably performed in six out of 44 X-ray images because of the partially visible femoral heads in two cases, and ambiguities in the determination of the center and inclination of the S1 endplate in four cases. As a result, these images were excluded from statistical comparison, which was in the end performed for images of 38 subjects (15 males/23 females; mean age 71.1 years, age range 49–85 years). The results are presented in terms of the mean absolute difference (MAD), the corresponding SD and the Pearson correlation coefficient ($R$). Statistical significance was observed through the paired $t$-test, with the level of significance set to $p < 0.05$.

Reference manual measurements amounted to $54.4 \pm 11.8°$ (mean $\pm$ SD) for PI, $35.0 \pm 8.7°$ for SS and $19.4 \pm 8.5°$ for PT, which is in accordance with existing population studies [2]. With the described fully automated approach we then successfully measured the same parameters, which amounted to $54.0 \pm 10.4°$ for PI, $34.3 \pm 8.6°$ for SS and $19.6 \pm 8.5°$ for PT. Statistical analysis of the agreement between manual and automated measurements is presented in Table 1 and Fig. 3.

**Table 1.** Statistical comparison between reference manual and fully automated measurements of pelvic incidence (PI), sacral slope (SS) and pelvic tilt (PT) from X-ray images of the pelvis of 38 subjects in terms of the mean absolute difference (MAD), standard deviation (SD), Pearson correlation coefficient ($R$), and $p$-value of the paired $t$-test.

|  | Pelvic incidence (PI) | Sacral slope (SS) | Pelvic tilt (PT) |
|---|---|---|---|
| MAD $\pm$ SD (°) | $5.1 \pm 4.4$ | $5.2 \pm 3.8$ | $2.2 \pm 2.0$ |
| $R$ ($p$-value) | $0.82\ (<10^{-6})$ | $0.73\ (<10^{-6})$ | $0.94\ (<10^{-6})$ |
| Paired $t$-test ($p$-value) | $0.691$ | $0.519$ | $0.627$ |

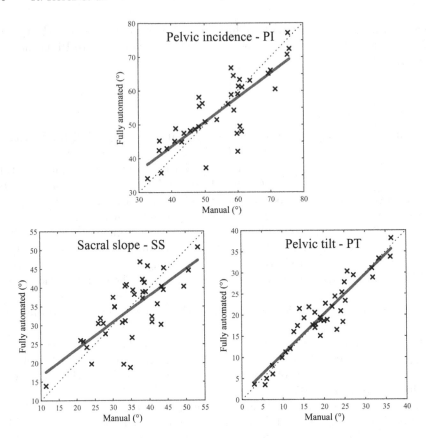

**Fig. 3.** Agreement between the manual and fully automated measurements.

## 4   Discussion

The determination of PI from X-ray images is a relatively demanding process because the projective nature of X-ray imaging causes a virtual superposition of the anatomical structures of interest. Moreover, different characteristics that originate from the natural biological variability of the human anatomy may also introduce ambiguities in the measurement process. Software packages that allow for computerized measurement of PI by manually drawing geometrical constructs (e.g. points, lines, circles) [4,7–10] proved to be more reproducible and reliable than measurements from plain X-ray films, as Vialle et al. [7] reported a mean reproducibility of $R = 0.86$ ($p = 0.014$) and $R = 0.96$ ($p < 0.001$), and a mean reliability of $R = 0.65$ ($p = 0.024$) and $R = 0.99$ ($p<0.001$) respectively for manual measurements of PI from plain X-ray films and digital X-ray images. Dimar II et al. [8] reported an even worse agreement, as they obtained a mean reproducibility of $R = 0.65$, 0.71 and 0.55 and a mean reliability of $R = 0.29$, 0.61 and 0.44 respectively for PI, SS and PT, while the agreement with computerized measurements was estimated to $R = 0.59$, 0.72 and 0.63, respectively.

Although computerized approaches improved the reproducibility and reliability, the measurement itself remains a relatively time-consuming and subjective task that highly depends on the experience of the observer. On the other hand, a fully automated measurement approach has not been yet presented, mostly because it represents a challenging problem from the perspective of automated analysis of X-ray images.

The described approach solves, to a certain degree, the afore mentioned problem. Statistical analysis (Table 1) revealed that there are no statistically significant differences between reference manual and fully automated measurements of PI, as well as of SS and PT. We can also conclude that the fully automated measurements are in agreement with reference manual measurements in the reliability range of classical and computerized manual measurements [7,8], as the correlation was good $(0.7 < R < 0.9)$ in the case of PI and SS, and very good $(0.9 < R < 1.0)$ in the case of PT. Nevertheless, high correlation and a relatively low MAD do not necessarily mean that the fully automated measurements are correct, moreover, a difference of around $5°$ may originate from the reproducibility and reliability of manual measurements [2]. The high agreement of reference manual and fully automated measurements results from applying the state-of-the-art deep learning technologies. It is also important to note that the proposed approach does not make use of already implemented techniques, but is refined with a detailed knowledge of CNN architectures, corresponding criterion functions and methods of supervised learning, as well as a detailed knowledge of spine and pelvis anatomy, and measurement of geometrical parameters from medical images.

## 5   Conclusion

In this paper, we presented the results of a fully automated measurement of PI from sagittal X-ray images of the pelvis. The results indicate that by this approach, it is possible to accurately determine PI, as the differences against reference manual measurements were within the range of the reproducibility and reliability of manual measurements. Nevertheless, the proposed fully automated approach cannot completely replace the visual review and confirmation of the measured values by an observer, as the differences may be in certain cases quite large, mostly due to the natural biological variability of the human anatomy and the characteristics induced by X-ray imaging.

**Acknowledgements.** This work was supported by Raylytic GmbH, Leipzig, Germany, partly by the Slovenian Research Agency under grants P2-0232 and J2-7118, and partly by the German Research Foundation (DFG) under project number PU 510/2-1.

# References

1. Duval-Beaupère, G., Schmidt, C., Cosson, P.: A Barycentremetric study of the sagittal shape of spine and pelvis: the conditions required for an economic standing position. Ann. Biomed. Eng. **20**(4), 451–462 (1992). https://doi.org/10.1007/BF02368136

2. Vrtovec, T., Janssen, M., Likar, B., Castelein, R., Viergever, M., Pernuš, F.: A review of methods for evaluating the quantitative parameters of sagittal pelvic alignment. Spine J. **12**(5), 433–446 (2012). https://doi.org/10.1016/j.spinee.2012.02.013

3. Le Huec, J., Aunoble, S., Leijssen, P., Pellet, N.: Pelvic parameters: origin and significance. Eur. Spine J. **20**(Suppl 5), S564–S571 (2011). https://doi.org/10.1007/s00586-011-1940-1

4. Berthonnaud, E., Labelle, H., Roussouly, P., Grimard, G., Vaz, G., Dimnet, J.: A variability study of computerized sagittal spinopelvic radiologic measurements of trunk balance. J. Spinal Disord. Tech. **18**(1), 66–71 (2005). https://doi.org/10.1097/01.bsd.0000128345.32521.43

5. Tyrakowski, M., Yu, H., Siemionow, K.: Pelvic incidence and pelvic tilt measurements using femoral heads or acetabular domes to identify centers of the hips: comparison of two methods. Eur. Spine J. **24**(1), 1259–1264 (2015). https://doi.org/10.1007/s00586-014-3739-3

6. Yamada, K., Aota, Y., Higashi, T., Ishida, K., Numura, T., Saito, T.: Accuracies in measuring spinopelvic parameters in full-spine lateral standing radiograph. Spine **40**(11), E640–E646 (2015). https://doi.org/10.1097/BRS.0000000000000904

7. Vialle, R., Ilharreborde, B., Dauzac, C., Guigui, P.: Intra and inter-observer reliability of determining degree of pelvic incidence in high-grade spondylolisthesis using a computer assisted method. Eur. Spine J. **15**(10), 1449–1453 (2006). https://doi.org/10.1007/s00586-006-0096-x

8. Dimar II, J., Carreon, L., Labelle, H., Djurasovic, M., Weidenbaum, M., Brown, C., et al.: Intra- and inter-observer reliability of determining radiographic sagittal parameters of the spine and pelvis using a manual and a computer-assisted methods. Eur. Spine J. **17**(10), 1373–1379 (2008). https://doi.org/10.1007/s00586-008-0755-1

9. Lafage, R., Ferrero, E., Henry, J., Challier, V., Diebo, B., Liabaud, B., et al.: Validation of a new computer-assisted tool to measure spino-pelvic parameters. Spine J. **15**(12), 2493–2502 (2015). https://doi.org/10.1016/j.spinee.2015.08.067

10. Maillot, C., Ferrero, E., Fort, D., Heyberger, C., Le Huec, J.C.: Reproducibility and repeatability of a new computerized software for sagittal spinopelvic and scoliosis curvature radiologic measurements: Keops®. Eur. Spine J. **24**(7), 1574–1581 (2015). https://doi.org/10.1007/s00586-015-3817-1

11. Lin, T., Goyal, P., Girshick, R., He, K., Dollár, P.: Focal loss for dense object detection. In: Proceedings of the IEEE International Conference on Computer Vision, ICCV 2017, pp. 2999–3007. IEEE (2017). https://doi.org/10.1109/ICCV.2017.324

12. Krizhevsky, A., Sutskever, I., Hinton, G.: ImageNet classification with deep convolutional neural networks. In: Pereira, F., et al. (eds.) Proceedings of the Neural Information Processing Systems, NIPS 2012, vol. 25, pp. 1097–1105. NIPS (2012)

# Author Index

Printed in the United States
By Bookmasters